MW01600180

GUT HEALTH SOLUTION

By
Health Coach Chris D. Henry

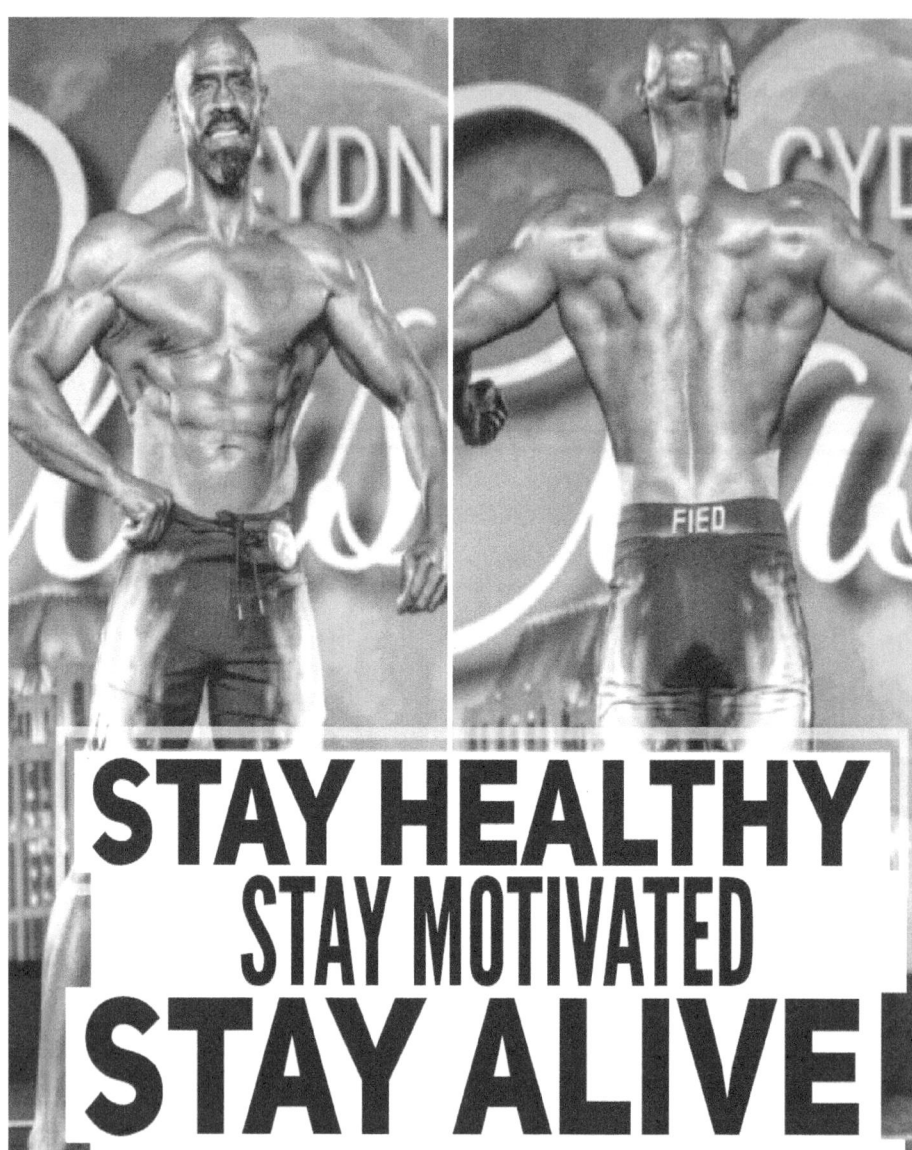

STAY HEALTHY
STAY MOTIVATED
STAY ALIVE

Gut Health Solution Copyright © 2024 by Chris Henry All rights reserved.

No part of this publication may be reproduced, distributed, or transmitted in any form or by any means, including photocopying, recording, or other electronic or mechanical methods, without the prior written permission of the publisher, except in the case of brief quotations embodied in critical reviews and certain other noncommercial uses permitted by copyright law. For permission requests, write to the publisher, addressed "Attention: Permissions Coordinator," at the address below.

Transform your health and wellness with "Gut Health Solution," a comprehensive guide to revitalizing your gut and enhancing your overall well-being.

Written by health coach Chris D. Henry, this essential resource unveils the secrets to achieving a healthier lifestyle through three simple yet powerful steps: Nutrition, Cardio, and Resistance Training. In this book, you'll discover how to make informed food choices that support your body's nutritional needs, enabling you to shed unwanted weight and maintain a resilient gut. Chris shares practical advice on what to eat, what to avoid, and how to reclaim your health in a world filled with unhealthy temptations.

Contents

CHAPTER 1

"Nourish to Flourish: Essential Health Tips for a Happy Gut"

It's crucial to understand the significant impact of our dietary choices on our health, especially today where unhealthy eating habits are prevalent. Many individuals find themselves struggling to lose weight, often overlooking the core issue: nutrition. If we aren't consuming the right foods, losing weight becomes a challenging game, while gaining it becomes all too easy. The alarming rise in health issues among the younger population, including cancer, high blood pressure, and heart-related illnesses, highlights a pressing concern.

Unfortunately, many people often rationalize their poor dietary choices with excuses. Statements like, "My partner is stressing me out," or "I don't have support," serve as justifications for opting for unhealthy foods. Moreover, as parents, we have a responsibility to be mindful of what we feed our children. Allowing unhealthy foods into their diets can have lasting consequences, impacting their overall health and wellness. We must take a proactive approach to educate ourselves and our families about the importance of good nutrition, setting an example that promotes healthier choices. That's why diabetes in children is at an all-time high in America.

Engaging in physical activity as a family is incredibly beneficial, and it's something that parents should prioritize. I have fond memories of my childhood when my father would insist that my brother and I play catch outside. When friends visited, he'd gather us all into a circle for a game, and then he'd humorously challenge us with, "Drop it and give me twenty!" We would all drop to the ground for push-ups, feeling like we were in some sort of boot camp. Those moments instilled in me the importance of staying active and fit from a young age.

Incorporating exercise into family time not only promotes health but also creates lasting memories and strengthens bonds. Making physical activity a fun part of our daily routine teaches children the value of exercise, setting them up for a lifetime of healthy habits. This kind of engagement can make fitness enjoyable, helping to instill a sense of discipline and teamwork, which are valuable lessons for any child.

As you embark on this new journey towards better health, the first step is to take a good look at your environment, specifically, your kitchen. It's time for a thorough cleanse! Begin by clearing out your refrigerator and kitchen cabinets of any unhealthy items. We all have a general understanding of what constitutes healthy and unhealthy foods, so there's no need to overthink it. Start your spring cleaning by tossing out all that junk food that might be tempting you. Say goodbye to those

Lays potato chips and other unhealthy snacks may often call to you with their irresistible crunch and flavor, but choosing healthier options is crucial for embarking on your wellness journey. Instead of using regular table salt, consider enhancing your dishes with alternatives like Himalayan salt or Mrs. Dash, both of which add a burst of flavor without compromising your health. Pink Himalayan salt is a treasure trove of beneficial minerals such as magnesium and calcium, which can have a profound impact on your overall well-being. By diligently removing unhealthy snacks from your kitchen and replacing them with nourishing alternatives, you're not just making a simple dietary change, you're establishing a strong, inspiring foundation for a lifetime of robust health and vitality!

The minerals in Himalayan salt are sulfate, magnesium, calcium, potassium, bicarbonate, bromide, borate, strontium, and fluoride (in descending order of quantity).

Because of these minerals Himalayan pink salt can:

- Create an electrolyte balance
- Increase hydration
- Regulate water content both inside and outside of cells
- Balance pH (alkaline/acidity) and help to reduce acid reflux
- Preventing muscle cramping
- Aid in proper metabolism functioning
- Strengthening bones
- Lower blood pressure

- Help the intestines absorb nutrients
- Prevent goiters
- Improve circulation
- Dissolve and eliminate sediment to remove toxins.

When considering healthy sources of protein, make baked and grilled skinless chicken, turkey, fish, and tofu your top choices. A practical approach is to dedicate some time on Sunday to grilling all your meats, ensuring that you have flavorful and nutritious meals prepared for the week ahead. If you don't already have a grill, consider purchasing one from your local grocery store or exploring sales at appliance retailers like Home Depot or Lowe's. To maintain a healthy lifestyle, it's important to avoid beef and pork, as these meats can contribute to high blood pressure and other health concerns.

Additionally, refraining from sweets and sugary drinks is essential, as they can significantly derail your progress. Staying well-hydrated by drinking plenty of water is equally vital, playing a crucial role in your weight loss journey. By prioritizing these healthier food choices, you will be establishing a strong foundation for your success!

Starting your day with a nutritious breakfast and including a healthy snack in between meals is crucial for kick-starting your metabolism. It's important not to delay your first meal until noon; eating in the morning fuels your body and sets the right tone for the day. Consider snacks like apples, grapes, protein shakes, bananas, peanuts, and smoothies—these options provide essential vitamins and minerals. Make sure to keep fruits and vegetables in your refrigerator or freezer, as they are packed with nutrients that aid in fat- burning and contribute to overall health. Incorporating these foods into your diet will help you not only control your weight but also maintain your energy levels throughout the day. Prioritizing these habits can significantly enhance your journey of wellness!

Brown rice and brown rice pasta are excellent sources of healthy carbohydrates that can enhance your overall wellness. It's essential to dispel the misconception that white starch is beneficial; options like white rice, white bread, white flour, and white pasta often lack the essential nutrients that support good health. Instead, consider adding baked potatoes to your meals, with sweet potatoes and purple potatoes being even better choices. Purple potatoes are especially advantageous as they help draw excess water from your body.

While they may be more readily available during the holiday season, you can also find them at specialty stores like Whole Foods, Fresh Market, or local farmers' markets. Making these thoughtful substitutions will aid in maintaining a healthier diet!

Absolutely NO sugary food! I REPEAT, "There shouldn't be any sugary drinks anywhere in your home!" Additionally, eliminate all unhealthy cooking oils, such as Crisco and other vegetable oils. If you enjoy baking, consider using whole wheat flour, specifically '100% Stone Ground, for making bread, muffins, pancakes, or other favorites, but I wouldn't recommend this until you've achieved your weight loss goals. This quick and easy guide is made to help you lose weight and sustain that loss effectively. You truly can transform your body into a fat-burning machine by training your muscles correctly. The key components are cardio, cardio, cardio, along with resistance training. If you have a gym membership or access to fitness equipment at home, you can embark on your journey today.

With over 15 years of experience training clients, I have observed a clear trend: those who demonstrate dedication and focus consistently achieve results, while those who lack commitment often encounter difficulties. Let's resolve not to start this year like those without motivation.

Instead, let's be the ones who take proactive steps and implement positive changes. Given the alarming increase in cancer and diabetes rates, prioritizing our health has never been more crucial; we must ensure we don't become part of those statistics. Let's embark on this journey together! If you have a treadmill or a cardio bike at home, begin using it now.

Pop in your favorite DVD or tune into your preferred television channel and start burning those calories right away.

Don't delay what you can accomplish today until tomorrow. This book aims to inspire you to act 'in the now.' Thus, as we enter this new year, let's eliminate any excuses! We will put an end to that mindset today with a clear goal in sight. So, what are you waiting for? I encourage you to start your workout routine as soon as you finish this book. No more excuses!

CHAPTER 2

"Move for Your Microbiome: Workouts to Boost Gut Health at Home and the Gym"

Focused on exercises that benefit digestive health, this chapter could include gentle home workouts, strength routines, and gym exercises to help reduce gut inflammation, improve circulation, and support a balanced gut.

When it comes to gut health, exercise might not be the first solution that comes to mind, yet it plays a vital role in maintaining a balanced microbiome and supporting digestive health. Physical activity has been shown to impact gut flora positively, aiding in the reduction of inflammation, improvement of circulation, and promotion of regular digestion. In this chapter, we'll explore how gentle home workouts, strength routines, and gym exercises can significantly impact your gut health. From gentle movements that are easy to do at home to structured routines you can do at the gym, each exercise is designed to encourage digestive health while contributing to your overall wellness.

Gentle Home Workouts for Gut Health

Starting with gentle, low-impact exercises can make a big difference, especially if you're new to regular physical activity or prefer working out at home. Movements like yoga, stretching, and walking are effective at reducing stress, which is key because high- stress levels can negatively impact the gut. For instance, yoga poses such as the "Cat-Cow," "Seated Twist," and "Child's Pose" stimulate the abdominal area, aiding in digestion and relieving bloating. Additionally, incorporating mindful breathing exercises alongside these poses can help your body switch to a relaxed, "rest-and-digest" mode, promoting smoother digestion. Walking after meals can also enhance gut motility, helping food move through the digestive tract more efficiently and preventing issues like gas and constipation.

Core-Strengthening Routines for Digestive Support

Core-focused exercises aren't just for building strength; they also provide significant digestive benefits. Engaging your core muscles helps support better posture, which improves abdominal pressure and reduces bloating and discomfort after meals. Exercises like planks, bicycle crunches, and Russian twists work not only to strengthen your abdominal muscles but also to massage and stimulate your digestive organs, encouraging regularity and relieving trapped gas. To maximize these benefits, consider incorporating core exercises into your workout routine at least three times a week, aiming for moderate reps to avoid over- straining. Building core strength is also excellent for posture, which plays a crucial role in allowing your internal organs to function without unnecessary pressure or constraint.

Full-Body Workouts and Cardiovascular Benefits for

the Gut

Cardiovascular exercises such as jogging, cycling, and swimming have been shown to boost circulation throughout the body, including the gut, helping deliver oxygen and nutrients more effectively to your digestive organs. Regular cardio can also assist in balancing gut bacteria, as studies show that active individuals tend to have a more diverse microbiome, a marker of a healthy gut. For a convenient approach, aim for 30 minutes of cardio a few times per week, even if it's brisk walking or a light jog around your neighborhood. Improved circulation from cardio exercises helps prevent digestive stagnation, allowing the digestive system to function more efficiently and supporting the absorption of nutrients. The positive impact of cardio extends to managing stress and reducing inflammation, both critical elements for a well-balanced gut.

Weightlifting for Better Gut Health

Weightlifting and resistance training may not seem directly connected to digestive health, but they offer surprising benefits. Strength training can aid in reducing systemic inflammation, which often originates in or affects the gut. Exercises like squats, deadlifts, and lunges work major muscle groups and encourage blood flow, which helps alleviate digestive issues like bloating and indigestion. For best results, start with lighter weights to avoid straining your core, and gradually increase as you build strength. Incorporating rest intervals between sets allows your body to process lactic acid, preventing the buildup that could otherwise contribute to muscle tension, which can disrupt digestion.

Weight training also supports better sleep and mood regulation, both of which contribute to gut health, making it an ideal addition to a balanced exercise routine.

Combining Mind and Body: Stress-Reducing Exercises for a Healthier Gut

Finally, combining stress-reducing techniques with your workouts can amplify gut health benefits. Exercises like tai chi and Pilates are not only gentle on the body but are also effective at calming the nervous system, which is crucial for managing stress. Tai chi, for example, involves slow, flowing movements that help calm the mind, reduce inflammation, and improve circulation throughout the body, including to your gut. Pilates, particularly focused on core strength and controlled breathing, aids in releasing tension in the abdominal area and encourages better digestion. By dedicating time to mind-body exercises a few times per week, you can reinforce a healthy gut-brain connection and contribute to a more balanced digestive system. Together, these approaches create a holistic movement plan that not only strengthens the body but also prioritizes gut health, setting a strong foundation for improved wellness overall.

To make your workout enjoyable, pop in your favorite DVD or turn on a show that you love, and then set your cardio machine for 25-35 minutes. If you feel up to it, feel free to go beyond that time! The more cardio you engage in and the more frequently you do it, the more efficiently your body will burn calories. After your workout, it's essential to replenish your body with a healthy smoothie or protein shake. This will help restore the minerals and nutrients you've expended during your exercise session.

Remember to stay hydrated by drinking plenty of water throughout the day; it's crucial for maintaining energy levels and supporting your overall health while you engage in cardio and resistance training. If you enjoy outdoor activities, dig out that bike that might be gathering dust in your garage and take it for a spin around your neighborhood. Just be sure that your area is safe for biking. Many newer communities have dedicated trails for walking and biking, making it easier to enjoy the outdoors while staying active!

I strongly encourage those who enjoy the outdoors to dust off their bikes and take them for a ride around the neighborhood. Before heading out, make sure that your area is safe for biking. Many modern communities feature trails designed for walking and biking, providing a great opportunity to enjoy nature while being active. For instance, in Atlanta, we have the Silver Comet Trail, which stretches through Cobb County, Douglas County, and all the way into Alabama. Stone Mountain Park is another favorite spot where people go jogging, walking, hiking, or biking. No matter where you live, it's important to find a community or park that meets your cardio needs. Aim for 3-5 days a week of some form of cardiovascular exercise to maintain a healthy and active lifestyle!

Boxing Class

Getting a boxing coach or taking any type of boxing class is great for people, especially women who are trying to lose fat behind their arms, or for people who are just trying to tone up their upper body.

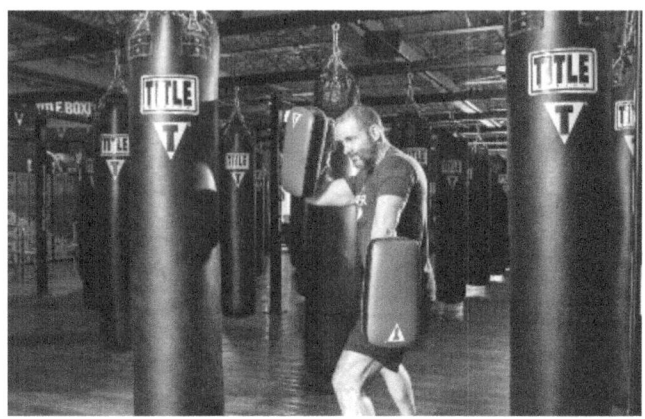

Resistance training is the key to losing fat and burning muscle. You can do cardio until you're blue in the face, but if you don't add any resistance training to your weekly workout, you won't see results like you'd hope to see. People who do too much cardio always tend to lose a lot of muscle during the process.

Over the years I have witnessed people who only come into the gym and run on the treadmill for about 45 minutes to an hour without getting muscle-building results. The reason is that they burn off too many calories and they're not putting those calories back into their bodies after they workout. This craziness happens repeatedly, and it can sometimes lead to high blood pressure and dizziness as well. People are known for passing out in the gym because of the lack of nutrients they have in their bodies.

Workout Recommendation

Beginners 3-4 sets of 12-15 reps

Advanced 5-7 sets of 15-25 reps

Step three - Resistance training

Resistance training plays a crucial role in building strength and improving overall fitness. Let's focus on a total body workout that incorporates some effective exercises. For chest workouts, consider performing push-ups, dumbbell chest presses, and straight bar chest presses. Additionally, cable or dumbbell flies and crossovers can help develop your chest muscles effectively.

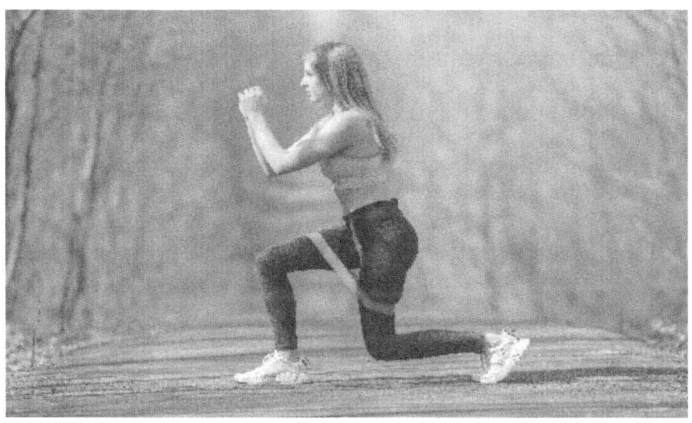

Resistance bands come in different levels of resistance, making them suitable for all fitness levels. They can be used for a wide range of exercises targeting various muscle groups, from arms and legs to core and back. These bands are lightweight and compact, making them easy to transport. You can use them at home, in the gym, or even while traveling, allowing you to maintain your workout routine anywhere.

Resistance bands provide a low-impact alternative to traditional weights, reducing the strain on your joints. This makes them an excellent option for individuals with joint issues or those recovering from injuries. Improved Stability and Balance. Because resistance bands require you to engage your core and stabilize your body during exercises, they help improve overall balance, coordination, and functional strength.

Bands allow for gradual increases in resistance. As you get stronger, you can switch to bands with higher resistance or increase the length of the band for more challenge. This progressive resistance plays a crucial role in muscle growth. Engagement of Stabilizing Muscles. When using resistance bands, your body must work harder to stabilize during movements. This engagement of stabilizing muscles can lead to better overall functional strength.

Note: You-Tube has videos that will show you the proper form for this particular exercise.

Beginners Pushups:

Beginners 3-4 sets of 5-10 reps

Advanced 5-7 sets of 15-25 reps

Using this easy push-up exercise will definitely build your upper body strength while grooming your push-up form as well. Make sure you're maintaining the proper form. This is perfect for beginners.

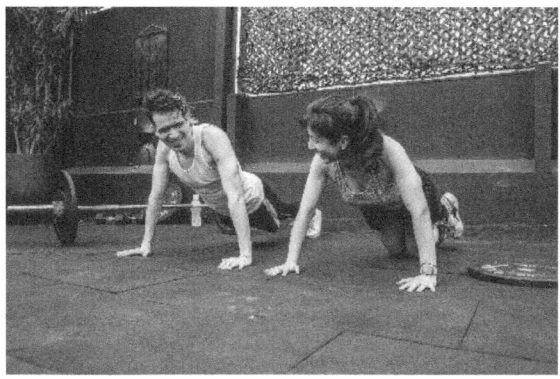

Note: You-Tube has videos that will show you the proper form for this particular exercise.

Regular Push-ups:

Beginners 3-4 sets of 12-15 reps

Advanced 5-7 sets of 15-25 reps

Make sure you're always keeping your back straight. Take at least 3 to 4-minute breaks in between your sets. You can also super-set this with abdominal exercises.

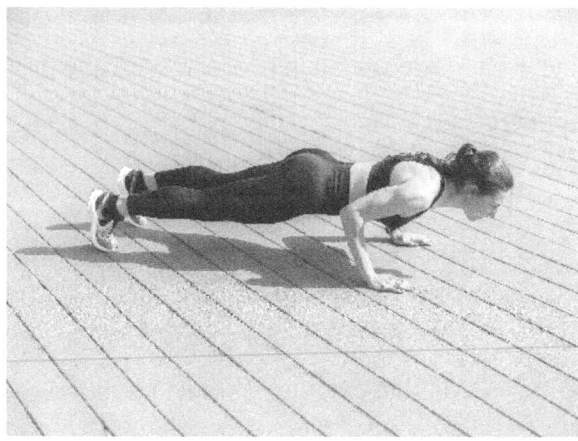

Note: You-Tube has videos that will show you the proper form for this particular exercise.

Elevated Push-ups:

Beginners 3-4 sets of 12-15 reps

Advanced 5-7 sets of 15-25 reps

This is a very advanced position. Make sure your hips don't drop as you go up and down doing this exercise. This exercise can really build your chest, shoulders, triceps, back, and core muscles. You can even super-set this with jumping jacks, jump ropes, or the running-in-place position.

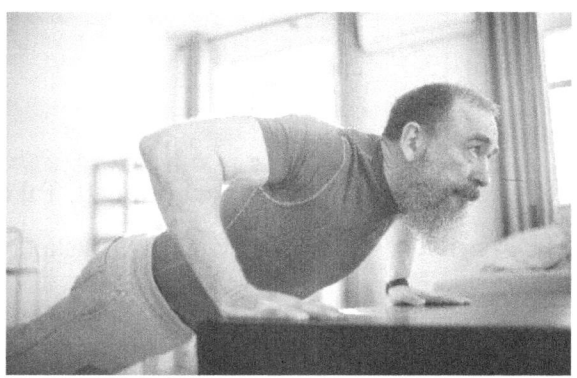

Note: You-Tube has videos that will show you the proper form for this particular exercise.

Push-ups on the Medicine Ball:

Beginners 3-4 sets of 12-15 reps

Advanced 5-7 sets of 15-25 reps

Beginners of this particular exercise should be able to do a regular push-up about 12 to 20 times per set before attempting this particular exercise. This is a great chest, back, shoulder, triceps, bicep and core exercise.

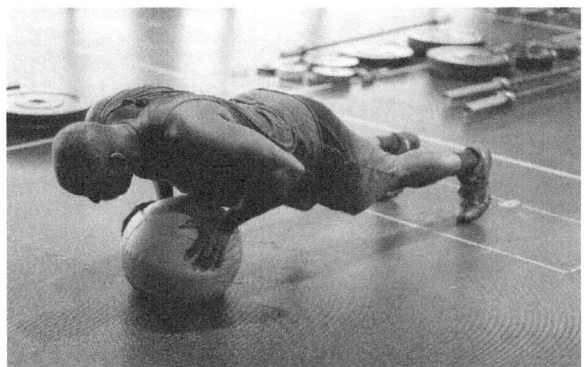

You can even hold your arms straight at the starting position for about 30 seconds to work your abdominal muscles as well (That particular position is called a straight arm plank).

Note: You-Tube has videos that will show you the proper form for this particular exercise.

Dumbbell Chest Press:

Beginners 3-4 sets of 12-15 reps

Advanced 5-7 sets of 15-25 reps

Make sure you squeeze your chest muscles once you extend your arms at the top. Your arms only need to go straight up and down. If you find your arms going all over the place, then drop the weight to an easier and more manageable weight.

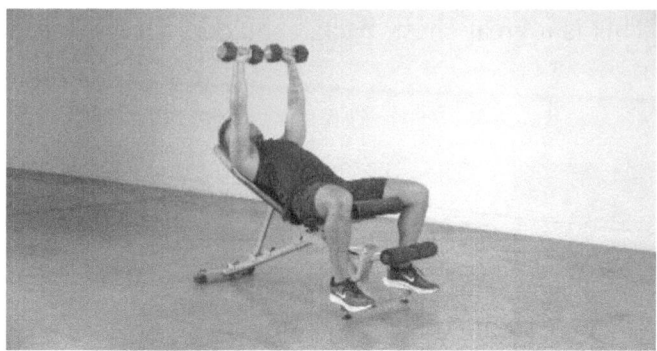

This exercise is great for toning and building your chest. It's all about consistency when you're doing all of these exercises.

Note: You-Tube has videos that will show you the proper form for this particular exercise.

Dumbbell flies lying on the floor:

Beginners 3-4 sets of 12-15 reps

Advanced 5-7 sets of 15-25 reps

Make sure your lower back stays flat and your legs stay in the upward position while your knees stay bent. This is great for building your chest muscles and your core muscles.

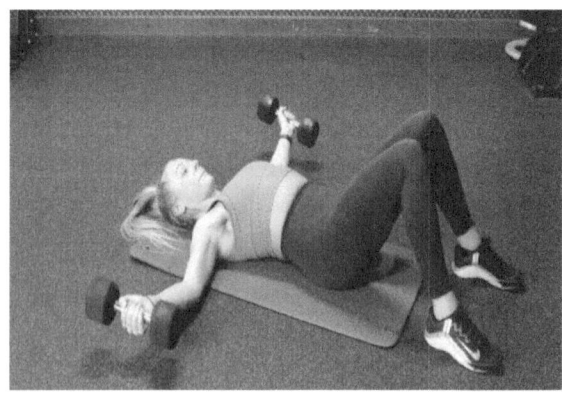

Note: You-Tube has videos that will show you the proper form for this particular exercise.

Cable Flies:

Beginners 3-4 sets of 12-15 reps

Advanced 5-7 sets of 15-25 reps

This is a great chest exercise for people who are trying to get that line in the middle of their chest. It's great for building your shoulder muscles as well. I recommend super setting this with flat bench chest presses every single time you're working your chest.

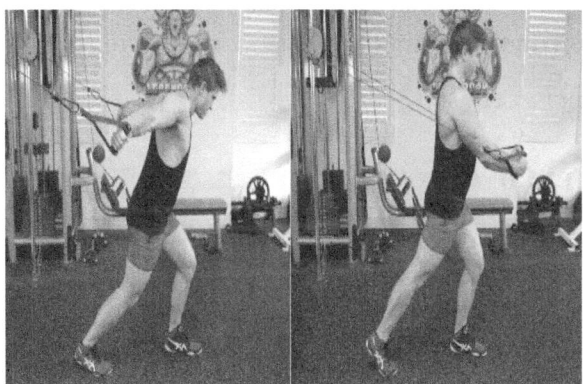

Note: You-Tube has videos that will show you the proper form for this particular exercise.

Bent over row extension:

Beginners 3-4 sets of 12-15 reps

Advanced 5-7 sets of 15-25 reps

This particular exercise is great for building your upper back muscles. Make sure you're keeping your back straight at all times. You can turn your hand in a palm-straight position or turn the dumbbell to a straight position so that it can line up with the bench. Either way is okay.

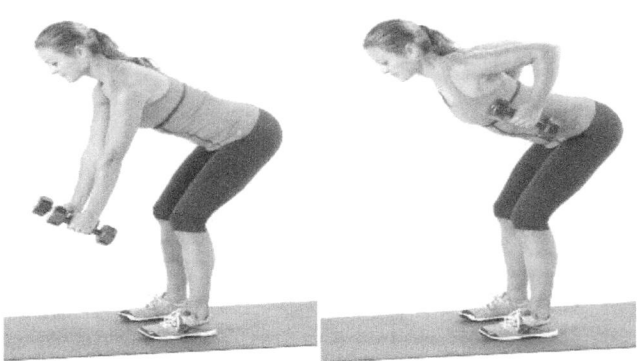

Note: You-Tube has videos that will show you the proper form for this particular exercise.

Barbell bent over row:

Beginners 3-4 sets of 12-15 reps

Advanced 5-7 sets of 15-25 reps

This particular back exercise is great for building your mid and lower back muscles. Once you bring your muscles up to your core, contract and squeeze your back muscles to get better results.

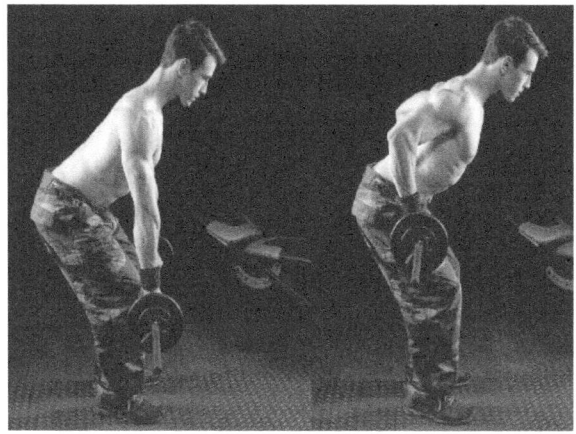

Note: You-Tube has videos that will show you the proper form for this particular exercise.

Behind the head Lat-pull:

Beginners 3-4 sets of 12-15 reps

Advanced 5-7 sets of 15-25 reps

I use this particular exercise to build my upper back muscles and my trapezius muscles. If done consistently, you'll see the benefits of this great exercise.

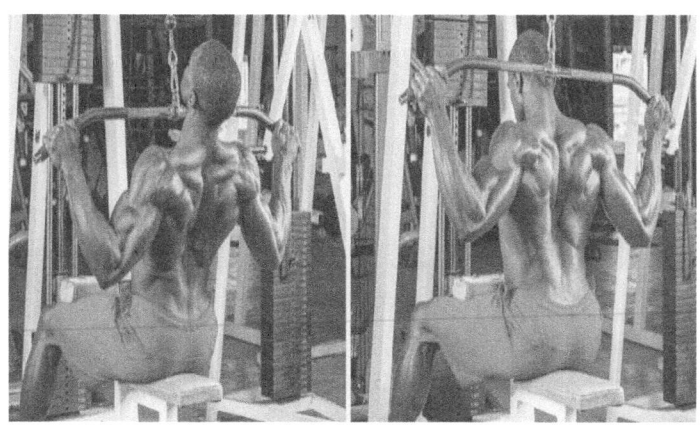

Note: You-Tube has videos that will show you the proper form for this particular exercise.

Dumbbell Shoulder Press:

Beginners 3-4 sets of 12-15 reps

Advanced 5-7 sets of 15-25 reps

Make sure you come down at a 45-degree angle. Taking your elbows lower than a 45-degree angle isn't a smart thing to do. We want to keep less stress off of the rotator cuff as much as possible. As long as you're doing this exercise correctly, you'll see great results.

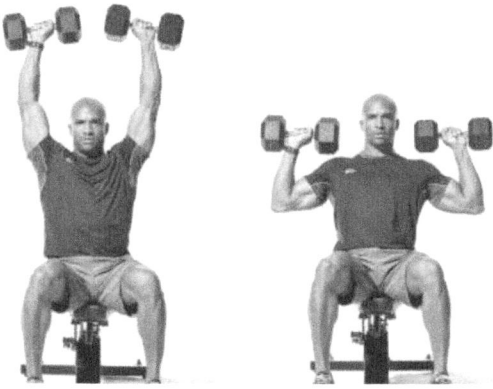

Note: You-Tube has videos that will show you the proper form for this particular exercise.

Bicep Barbell Curls:

Beginners 3-4 sets of 12-15 reps

Advanced 5-7 sets of 15-25 reps

Keep your body in line and don't bend your back while doing this particular exercise. Keep your back straight at all times. Squeeze your biceps at the top once you bring the weight up. I recommend doing this particular exercise three times a week.

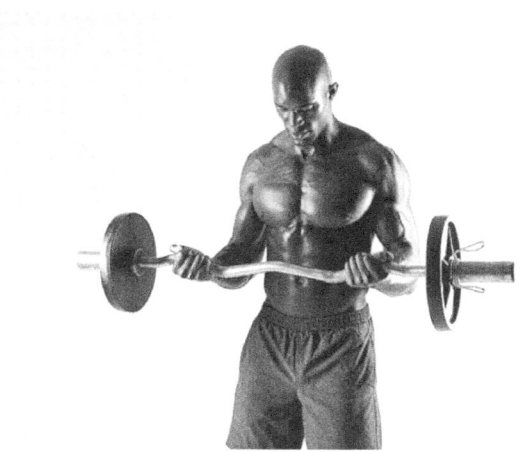

Note: You-Tube has videos that will show you the proper form for this particular exercise.

Triceps Rope Push-Downs:

Beginners 3-4 sets of 12-15 reps

Advanced 5-7 sets of 15-25 reps

Triceps extensions using the straight bar or the rope, are very effective as well. Make sure your form is correct while doing this particular exercise. Squeeze your triceps at the endpoint to get better results. I recommend doing this exercise at least 3 times a week for maximum results.

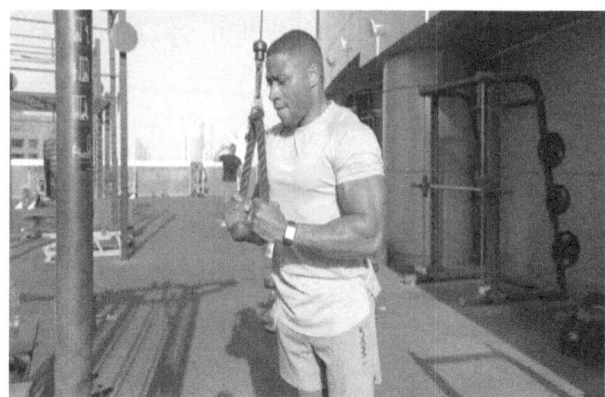

Note: You-Tube has videos that will show you the proper form for this particular exercise.

Sumo Squat:

Beginners 3-4 sets of 12-15 reps

Advanced 5-7 sets of 15-25 reps

Ladies looking to tone up their glutes and hamstrings should do this particular exercise. Hold your position at the endpoint for about 2 seconds and squeeze your glutes once you come back up.

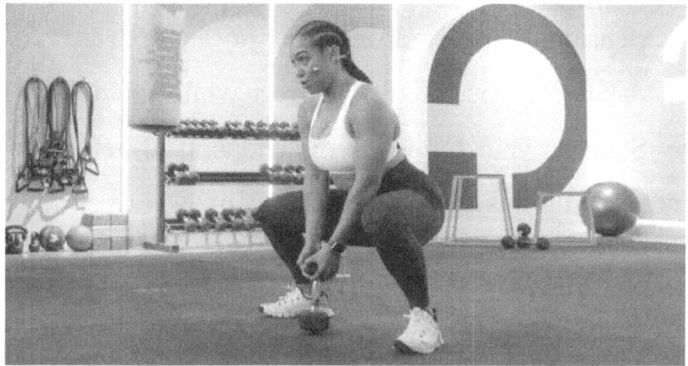

This is a simple leg exercise that you can do at home. I recommend this exercise at least twice a week. And three times a week for people who are more advanced.

Note: You-Tube has videos that will show you the proper form for this particular exercise.

Walking Lunges:

Beginners 3-4 sets of 12-15 reps

Advanced 5-7 sets of 15-25 reps

Lunges by far is my favorite leg exercise. You can do lunges in the gym, in your driveway at home, around your neighborhood, and at the local track as well. Lunges build your glutes, hamstrings, quads, and calves. Take advantage of this particular exercise whenever you have downtime. Advanced people can do lunges from 100 to 200 to 300 and even 400 meters. Do not attempt these types of distances if you're a beginner. Beginners just need to focus on short distances.

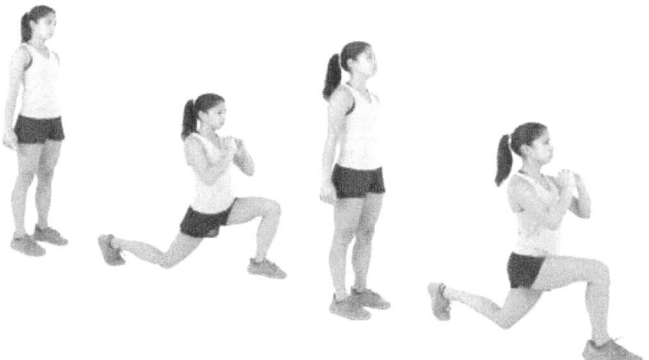

Using your driveway at home is a great place to start. The sidewalk in your neighborhood is a great place to start as well. I recommend beginners do lunges at least 15 to 20 yards.

Note: You-Tube has videos that will show you how to do lunges the correct way.

In Place Lunges:

Beginners 3-4 sets of 12-15 reps

Advanced 5-7 sets of 15-25 reps

Stationary lunges are great for beginners as well. Especially for mothers who are looking to get back in shape. Once you go forward, plant your feet down, and do not allow your knee to go past your toes. Make sure you extend your leg out far enough so that your knee lines up with your toes.

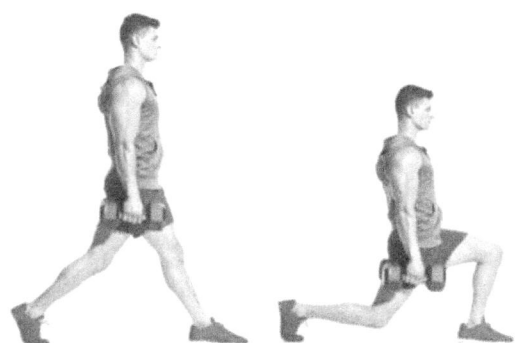

Note: There are several You-Tube videos you can check out as well.

Romanian Dead Lift:

Beginners 3-4 sets of 12-15 reps

Advanced 5-7 sets of 15-25 reps

Keep your knees slightly bent doing this exercise. Focus on working your glutes, hamstrings and lower back muscles. Make sure you do this particular exercise in a slow, upward and downward movement, while staying focused on the muscles you're working.

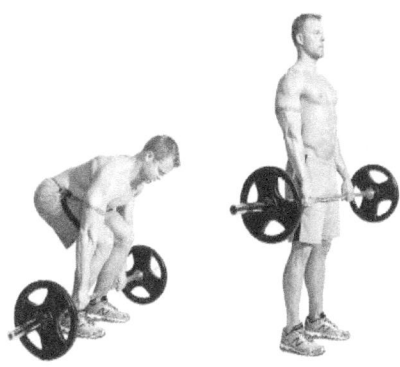

Note: There are several You-Tube videos you can check out as well.

Standing Calves Raises:

Beginners 3-4 sets of 15-25 reps

Advanced 5-7 sets of 25-40 reps

This is a simple exercise that you can do in the gym and at home. It takes hard work to build your calves. But when you're focused, determined, and dedicated to making your calves transform, you'll see results. Calves can be worked every day as well. Take advantage of this special and amazing exercise. Make sure you use the seated and standing calf machines at the gym you go to as well.

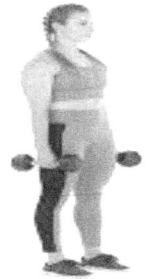 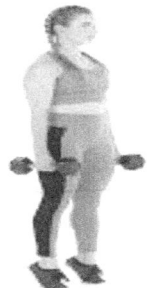

Note: You-Tube has videos that will show you how to do this exercise the correct way.

Ab Wheel Roll Out:

Beginners 3-4 sets of 12-15 reps

Advanced 5-7 sets of 15-25 reps

This is a game changer for everyone trying to lose body fat in their abdominal area. The ab wheel helps develop core, shoulders, arms, and back muscles. And the great thing about using the ab wheel is that you don't have to extend your arms out. Just extend your arms as far as you can and bring the wheel back to the starting position. You'll also see a change in your abs with this method. Just make sure you're using the ab wheel a few days a week. Abdominal muscles can be worked every day.

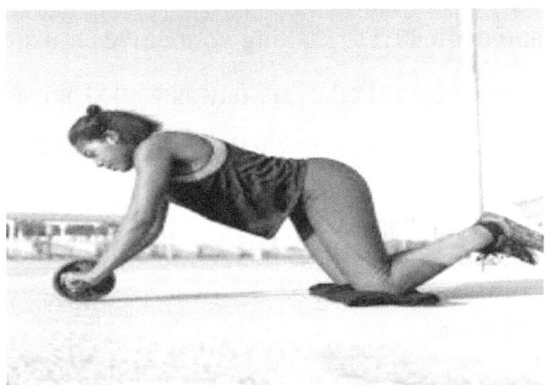

Note: You-Tube has videos that will show you how to do this exercise the correct way.

Crunches:

Beginners 3-4 sets of 12-15 reps

Advanced 5-7 sets of 15-25 reps

This is a basic ab exercise that's great when super-setting with the ab wheel and lying medicine ball twist. Keep your chin up facing the ceiling of the room. Don't over-strain your neck doing this particular exercise. I recommend anyone who's doing this exercise to super-set it with at least two more ab exercises for better results.

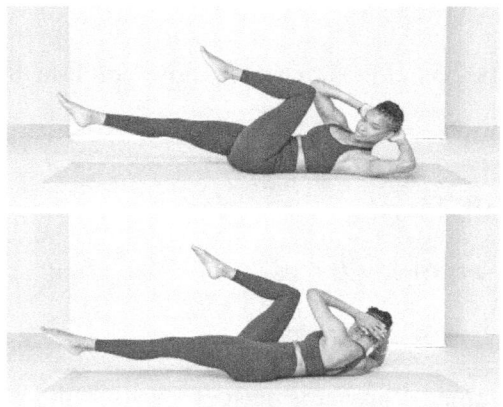

Note: You-Tube has videos that will show you how to do this exercise the correct way.

Side crunches:

Beginners 3-4 sets of 15-20 reps

Advanced 5-7 sets of 20-30 reps

Super-set this exercise with regular crunches, side bends (Page 33), the ab wheel, planks and bench kick-outs. Keep your head facing straight ahead and keep your chin up looking towards the ceiling while doing this exercise. This is great for burning those love handles that so much of us complain about.

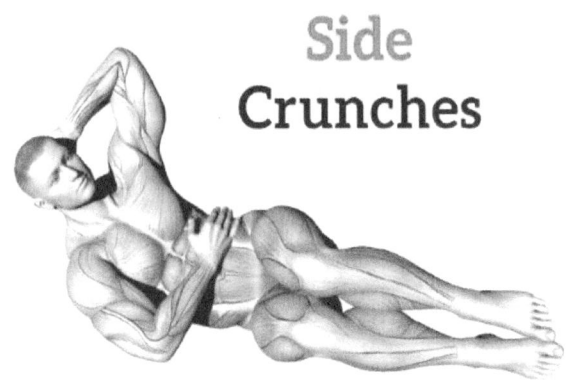

Note: You-Tube has videos that will show you how to do this exercise the correct way.

Medicine Ball Twist:

Beginners 3-4 sets of 15-20 reps

Advanced 5-7 sets of 20-30 reps

The lying medicine ball twist is perfect for your mid-core and your side core as well. This exercise can definitely help you with those love handles. Super-set this exercise with the ab wheel and crunches.

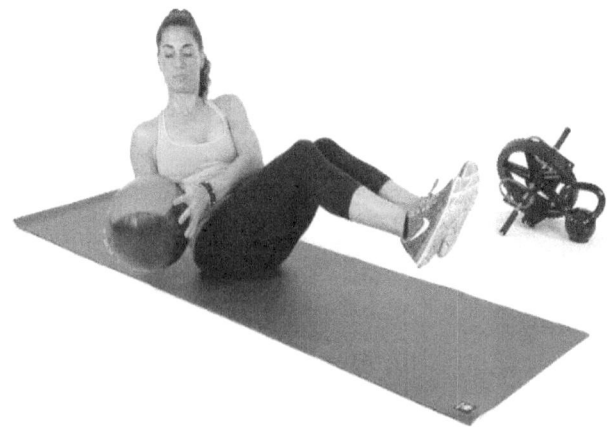

Note: YouTube has videos that will show you how to do this exercise the correct way.

Seated Flat Bench Leg kick outs:

Beginners 3-4 sets of 12-15 reps

Advanced 5-7 sets of 15-25 reps

This particular exercise is great for working your lower abs. If you have a weight bench at home, you can do this exercise at home.

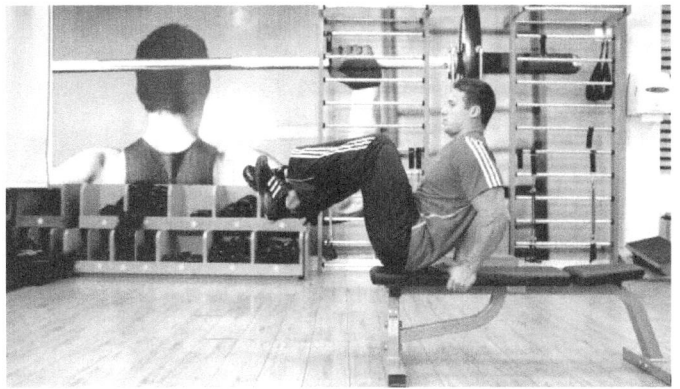

Note: Nutrition plays a major role in developing your abdominal muscles. I can't stress this important information enough. YOU, need to have a strict eating regimen in order to see the results you want to see.

Note: YouTube has videos that will show you how to do this exercise the correct way.

Standing side bends:

Beginners 3-4 sets of 12-15 reps

Advanced 5-7 sets of 15-25 reps

Super-set this exercise with crunches, the ab wheel, planks, bench ab kickouts, etc. This is also great for getting rid of love handles as well.

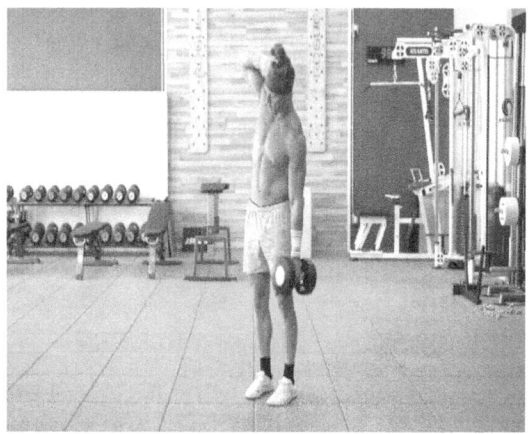

Note: YouTube has videos that will show you how to do this exercise the correct way.

CHAPTER 3

" Solutions for a Stronger Gut: Natural Remedies and Daily Practices"

This chapter could offer actionable gut health solutions, from probiotic-rich foods to lifestyle adjustments and simple, effective remedies for supporting and healing the gut microbiome.

The health of your gut is foundational to your overall wellness, impacting everything from digestion and nutrient absorption to immune function and mental well-being. To nurture a balanced microbiome, incorporating probiotic-rich foods, making mindful lifestyle adjustments, and using simple, effective remedies are key steps. In this chapter, we'll explore how these approaches can work together to support and heal the gut. By focusing on both diet and lifestyle, you can create a holistic foundation that promotes a healthier digestive system and contributes to a resilient, well-functioning gut microbiome.

Incorporating Probiotic-Rich Foods for Gut Balance

One of the most effective ways to support your gut microbiome is by incorporating probiotic-rich foods into your diet. Probiotics are beneficial bacteria that can help balance the natural flora in your gut, which is essential for maintaining good digestion and preventing the overgrowth of harmful bacteria. Foods like yogurt, kefir, sauerkraut, kimchi, and miso are rich sources of probiotics. Including a small serving of these foods daily can help maintain a healthy balance in your gut microbiome. For example, yogurt with live, active cultures is an easy and delicious way to boost your probiotic intake. Additionally, fermented vegetables like sauerkraut and kimchi not only provide beneficial bacteria but also contain fiber, which acts as a prebiotic, feeding the good bacteria and helping them thrive. Consuming these foods regularly can be a gentle yet powerful way to improve your gut health naturally.

Emphasizing Fiber-Rich, Prebiotic Foods to Fuel Good Bacteria

Alongside probiotics, it's crucial to consume enough prebiotics—types of fiber that feed the beneficial bacteria in your gut. Prebiotic foods include garlic, onions, leeks, asparagus, bananas, and oats. When these foods are broken down, they become fuel for the good bacteria in your gut, allowing them to multiply and maintain a balanced microbiome.

By supporting the probiotics in your system, prebiotics act as a foundation for gut health, promoting better digestion, nutrient absorption, and overall wellness. For instance, incorporating a banana or a serving of oats into your morning routine can be an easy way to boost prebiotic intake without extra effort. The combination of prebiotics and probiotics, often called "synbiotics," can be incredibly effective in promoting a balanced, healthy gut environment.

Making Mindful Lifestyle Adjustments for Better Gut Health

Lifestyle plays a crucial role in gut health, with factors like sleep, stress management, and hydration all affecting the microbiome. Prioritizing good-quality sleep is essential, as insufficient sleep can disrupt the balance of gut bacteria and increase inflammation. Aim to establish a regular sleep routine to allow your body the time it needs to repair and rejuvenate. Stress management is equally important, as chronic stress can lead to an imbalance in gut bacteria, often called dysbiosis, and may impair digestion. Practices such as meditation, deep breathing, and regular physical activity can help mitigate stress, promoting a healthier gut environment. Staying well-hydrated also aids digestion by helping food move smoothly through the intestines, which supports regular bowel movements and prevents constipation. By addressing these aspects of your lifestyle, you can create an environment that's conducive to gut health and overall wellness.

Using Natural Remedies to Soothe Digestive Discomfort

Sometimes, natural remedies can offer quick relief for common digestive discomforts like bloating, gas, and indigestion. Ingredients such as ginger, peppermint, and chamomile are known for their soothing effects on the digestive tract. For example, ginger has natural anti-inflammatory properties that can help reduce nausea and improve digestion, while peppermint can relax the muscles in the gastrointestinal tract, relieving bloating and discomfort. Chamomile tea, often used as a mild sedative, can also soothe the gut and alleviate indigestion. Additionally, a small amount of apple cider vinegar mixed with water before meals can aid in stimulating stomach acid production, which helps break down food more effectively. These remedies are not only natural but also easy to incorporate into your daily routine, offering gentle yet effective ways to support your gut health and alleviate occasional digestive discomforts.

Developing a Consistent Gut Health Routine for Lasting Benefits

Creating a daily routine focused on gut health can reinforce all the dietary and lifestyle adjustments you're making. Consistency is key, as the gut microbiome responds well to stable, routine behaviors. Start by building small, manageable habits, such as incorporating probiotic and prebiotic foods into your meals, practicing regular physical activity, and taking time each day to de-stress.

Tracking your food intake and noting any reactions can also provide insights into which foods support or challenge your gut health. This routine can evolve as you learn what works best for you, creating a sustainable approach to gut health. Over time, these practices will not only support a balanced gut but also contribute to enhanced immunity, improved energy levels, and better overall health.

Chlorophyll:

Incorporating chlorophyll into your nightly routine can be a game-changer for your metabolism! This powerful natural supplement is readily available at your local Vitamin Shoppe or can be conveniently ordered online. Chlorophyll is a fantastic fat-soluble compound that helps effectively burn body fat. For optimal results, simply add a teaspoon of chlorophyll to your 16oz water bottle, drinking one serving in the morning and another at night.

Not only does chlorophyll aid in alkalizing your body, but it also has cancer-fighting properties, making it an essential addition to your health regimen. Don't miss out on this must-have supplement that everyone should consider for a healthier lifestyle!

This supplement is a must-have for anyone seriously invested in their health and wellness journey. Whether you're looking to improve digestion, boost energy levels, or simply support your immune system, incorporating chlorophyll into your daily routine could be a transformative step toward a healthier lifestyle.

Don't overlook the potential benefits—make chlorophyll a staple in your wellness toolkit today

Baking Soda:

Baking soda is an incredibly versatile substance, offering a range of health benefits that can support your overall well-being. One notable advantage is its ability to help alkalize your body. Simply add a pinch of baking soda to your bottled water and drink it in the morning and at night. This practice can improve bowel movements and promote skin health by cleansing from within. Even professional swimmers incorporate baking soda into their routines to enhance performance and timing.

By providing the body with oxygen, baking soda aids in better respiration. But that's not all; it has also been linked to various health benefits, including potentially combating cancerous diseases. When introducing baking soda to your regimen, it's advisable to use it for the first seven days, then take a five-day break. After that, consider using it every other day to avoid over-alkalizing your body.

In addition to baking soda, consider incorporating chlorophyll into your daily routine. Chlorophyll is a

powerful liquid supplement that can work harmoniously with baking soda to support your health. I use both regularly and highly recommend them for their combined benefits!

Aloe Vera Gel:

Aloe vera gel is renowned for its numerous health and beauty benefits, making it a popular choice for many. Here are some of the key advantages:

1. Aloe vera gel is famous for its ability to soothe sunburn and other skin irritations. Its anti- inflammatory properties help reduce redness and promote healing.
2. It acts as a natural moisturizer for the skin without leaving a greasy residue, making it suitable for all skin types. Its hydrating properties help keep skin soft and supple.
3. Aloe vera can accelerate the healing process of minor cuts,

burns, and abrasions. Its antibacterial properties also help prevent infections.

4. The antioxidants, vitamins, and enzymes in aloe vera can help reduce the appearance of fine lines and wrinkles, promoting a more youthful

5. complexion.

6. Aloe vera gel has antimicrobial properties that can help reduce acne and prevent breakouts. It also soothes inflamed skin and helps reduce scarring.

7. When consumed, aloe vera can support digestive health by aiding digestion and reducing symptoms of constipation. It is believed to balance gut flora.

8. Aloe vera gel is a good source of hydration. Drinking aloe vera juice can help maintain hydration levels in the body.

9. Aloe vera contains vitamins, minerals, and antioxidants that may help support the immune system and improve overall wellness.

10. It can be used as a natural conditioner, helping to hydrate and nourish the scalp while reducing dandruff and promoting hair growth.

11. Aloe vera gel can be used in oral care products to promote healthier gums and reduce plaque.

By incorporating aloe vera gel into your skincare routine or diet, you can enjoy these benefits, making it a valuable addition to your health and wellness arsenal. Always remember to do a patch test when using it on your skin and consult with a healthcare professional if you're considering taking it internally.

Health Benefits

- Supports healthy digestion
- Supports a healthy immune system
- Reduces harmful toxins
- Increases absorption of nutrients
- Enhances antioxidant support
- Balances stomach acidity naturally
- Soothes occasional muscle and joint discomfort

Ancient Aztec Super Food Chia Seeds:

Chia seeds are great for protein, omega-3, iron, calcium, etc. They have three times more anti-oxidants than blueberries, are gluten-free, and are great for vegetarians and vegans. Chia seeds are a great substitute for protein if you don't like drinking protein shakes. If you're having problems with high blood pressure and your cholesterol, chia seeds will help lower the levels of both your high blood pressure and cholesterol.

Once you start taking chia seeds, make sure you're monitoring your high blood pressure by checking it every week.

There are Pharmacy stores and Grocery stores that have areas set up for you to sit down and self- check your blood pressure.

You can add two tablespoons of chia seeds to a gallon of water, or you can add one tablespoon to a 16 oz bottle of water as well. Once added, shake the bottle or jug so that the chia seeds can spread around inside the bottle or jug. Allow the chia seeds to soak in the water for about 20 to 25 minutes and then drink and

enjoy.

Here are some key advantages:

1. Chia seeds are a rich source of essential nutrients, including fiber, protein, healthy fats, vitamins, and minerals.
2. They contain a significant amount of alpha- linolenic acid (ALA), a plant-based omega-3 fatty acid that supports heart health.
3. Chia seeds are loaded with antioxidants that help protect the body from oxidative stress and free radical damage.
4. Their high fiber content promotes regular bowel movements, supports gut health, and helps maintain a healthy digestive system.
5. When soaked in water, chia seeds absorb up to
6. 12 times their weight, creating a gel-like substance that aids in hydration and can help you feel full.
7. The combination of protein, fiber, and gel- forming properties can help you feel satiated, making it easier to manage hunger and support weight loss.
8. Chia seeds may improve insulin sensitivity and help stabilize blood sugar levels, which is beneficial for individuals with diabetes.
9. They are rich in calcium, phosphorus, magnesium, and other vital nutrients that contribute to bone strength and overall

skeletal health.

10. The fiber, omega-3 fatty acids, and antioxidants in chia seeds can help lower cholesterol levels and reduce inflammation, promoting cardiovascular health.

11. Chia seeds can be easily incorporated into various dishes, including smoothies, yogurt, salads, and baked goods, making them a versatile addition to any diet. Incorporating chia seeds into your daily routine can provide numerous health benefits, contributing to

12. overall wellness and vitality. Whether used in recipes or as a supplement, these tiny seeds can make a big impact on your health!

Foods that Boost your Metabolism

1. Eggs – Eggs jump starts your morning and kick off your metabolism to help burn fat throughout the day.

2. Chia Seeds - A mere tablespoon of this powerful plant food packs a walloping 2,500 milligrams of omega-3 fatty acids, 4.5 grams of fiber, three grams of protein, and a boatload of phytonutrients.

3. Cinnamon is a fat-burning powerhouse that helps boost your metabolism. It is also proven to help your body block the absorption of glucose and enhance the action of insulin to clear sugar from your blood.

4. Berries - Studies suggest these compounds reduce body weight gain, inhibit fat accumulation, possess anti-inflammatory and

anti-diabetic properties, and alter gut flora to inhibit the growth of harmful pathogens.

5. Ginger – This popular and amazing spice helps

6. ease hunger, increases fat burn, and can be used as a home remedy to help ease symptoms of digestive complaints, including constipation, dyspepsia, belching, bloating, epigastric discomfort, indigestion, and nausea.

7. Green Tea - Green tea's caffeine enhances energy expenditure and fat oxidation by activating the sympathetic nervous system, while the polyphenols counteract the reflex decrease in the resting metabolic rate that usually accompanies weight loss.

8. Avocado - Avocado oil is especially high in monounsaturated fatty acids (MUFAs), including an omega-9 fat called oleic acid—a MUFA that has been shown to quiet hunger. MUFA-rich diets also protect against abdominal fat.

9. Quinoa - Gluten-free quinoa is high in magnesium, which is a key regulator of energy and promotes good blood sugar control.

10. Cayenne - When eating Cayenne peppers, your

11. sympathetic nervous system (also known as the fight-or-flight response) is activated, and hormones called catecholamines—such as epinephrine and norepinephrine—are released into the bloodstream. This process increases thermogenesis, whereby fat is oxidized more effectively. That means you are fat becomes fuel for your metabolic fire in as few as 20 minutes after eating cayenne.

Note: Drinking Green Tea while working out can super boost your metabolism. This method is known for helping people burn fat twice as fast.

Organic Flour and Organic Coconut Oil:

It's not what you eat! It's how you prepare it. You can find whole wheat flour and coconut oil in grocery stores like Kroger's, Publix, Whole Foods, etc. Use these two great products if you want to prepare the following foods. Note: This is only a treat after you complete your three-month weight loss goal.

- Fried Chicken
- Cookies
- Bread
- Muffins
- Sweet Potato Fries/ Sauteed Veggies
- Bagels
- Fried Salmon
- Pizza Crust
- Pancakes
- Brownies

CHAPTER 4

" Understanding Gut Health, The Importance of Gut Health"

The health of the gut plays a fundamental role in overall well-being, significantly influencing various bodily functions, including digestion, metabolism, and immune response. A balanced gut flora is essential for optimal health, as it aids in nutrient absorption, regulates inflammation, and protects against harmful pathogens. In recent years, research has illuminated the intricate relationship between gut health and conditions such as obesity, diabetes, and even mental health disorders. For fitness and health enthusiasts, maintaining a healthy gut can enhance energy levels, improve athletic performance, and foster recovery, making it a critical focus in any wellness regimen.

Herbs and food are powerful allies in promoting gut health. Specific herbs, such as ginger, peppermint, and turmeric, possess anti-inflammatory and soothing properties that can alleviate digestive discomfort and enhance gut function. Incorporating these herbs into daily nutrition can help combat symptoms of digestive disorders, including irritable bowel syndrome (IBS) and bloating. Additionally, herbal teas infused with these ingredients can provide a gentle yet effective means of supporting digestive wellness, offering both hydration and therapeutic benefits.

Prebiotic foods are another vital component of gut health, serving as nourishment for beneficial gut bacteria. Foods rich in prebiotics, such as garlic, onions, bananas, and asparagus, can help balance gut flora, fostering an environment where beneficial bacteria thrive. This balance is crucial, as a diverse microbiome is associated with improved digestion and a strengthened immune system. For fitness enthusiasts, incorporating these foods into meals not only supports gut health but also enhances overall nutritional intake, providing essential vitamins and minerals required for peak performance.

Smoothies can serve as an excellent vehicle for gut-friendly ingredients, allowing for creative combinations that deliver maximum health benefits. By blending fruits, vegetables, and prebiotic foods with gut-supportive herbs, individuals can create nutrient-dense smoothies that promote digestive health. Ingredients like spinach, chia seeds, and probiotic-rich yogurt can be included to further boost gut flora balance. These smoothies not only provide essential nutrients but also offer a convenient and delicious way to incorporate gut-friendly foods into a busy lifestyle.

In addition to dietary changes, herbal remedies can play a significant role in addressing specific digestive disorders. For those experiencing chronic digestive issues, targeted herbal supplements can offer relief and support. Herbs such as fennel and chamomile are known for their calming effects on the digestive tract, while others like slippery elm can soothe irritation. By embracing a holistic approach that includes dietary adjustments, herbal solutions, and mindful practices, individuals can cultivate a healthier gut, ultimately enhancing their fitness journey and overall quality of life.

Common Gut Health Issues

Many individuals striving for optimal health encounter common gut health issues that can impede their progress. These issues often manifest as bloating, constipation, diarrhea, or abdominal discomfort, and they can significantly impact overall well-being. While various factors contribute to these problems, including stress and poor diet, an imbalance in gut flora frequently plays a pivotal role. Understanding these gut health issues is essential for devising effective strategies to promote digestive wellness and enhance fitness routines.

One prevalent gut health issue is Irritable Bowel Syndrome (IBS), a functional gastrointestinal disorder characterized by symptoms such as cramping, abdominal pain, and altered bowel habits. IBS can be exacerbated by certain foods, stress levels, and hormonal fluctuations. Incorporating anti-inflammatory herbs like ginger and turmeric into the diet can help alleviate symptoms by reducing inflammation in the gut. Additionally, herbal teas such as peppermint and chamomile offer soothing properties that may ease digestive discomfort, making them valuable allies for those managing IBS.

Another common concern is dysbiosis, an imbalance of gut bacteria that can lead to various digestive problems. This condition may result from antibiotic use, poor diet, or high-stress levels. To combat dysbiosis, the inclusion of prebiotic foods, such as garlic, onions, and bananas, is crucial as they nourish beneficial gut bacteria. Furthermore, fermented foods like yogurt and kefir can introduce live probiotics, promoting a balanced gut microbiome. Adopting a diet rich in these foods can support gut health and improve overall digestive function.

Constipation is another frequent issue that many health-conscious individuals face. This condition can be linked to inadequate fiber intake and dehydration. Herbal remedies, such as senna and flaxseed, can act as natural laxatives, providing relief. Moreover, incorporating high-fiber foods like whole grains, fruits, and vegetables into meals can enhance bowel regularity. Gut-friendly smoothies, made with ingredients like spinach, chia seeds, and almond milk, not only provide hydration but also deliver essential nutrients that support digestive health.

Lastly, chronic inflammation in the gut can lead to more severe health issues over time, including autoimmune disorders. Anti-inflammatory herbs, such as boswellia and licorice root, may help mitigate this inflammation and promote healing in the digestive tract. Regularly consuming detoxifying herbs like dandelion and burdock root can also support liver function and aid in cleansing the gut. By being proactive and incorporating these herbal solutions and dietary adjustments, fitness and health enthusiasts can effectively tackle common gut health issues, paving the way for improved overall well-being and enhanced physical performance.

How Herbs and Foods Impact the Gut

The relationship between herbs, foods, and gut health is a vital aspect of overall wellness that fitness and health enthusiasts should prioritize. Our gut plays a crucial role in digestion, nutrient absorption, and immune function. Incorporating specific herbs and foods can significantly influence the gut microbiome, the community of microorganisms that reside in our digestive tract. These microorganisms are essential for maintaining a balanced gut environment, and the right dietary choices can promote their health and diversity. Understanding how these natural elements interact with our digestive system can empower individuals to make informed decisions for optimal gut health.

Herbs such as ginger, peppermint, and chamomile have long been recognized for their digestive benefits. Ginger, known for its anti-inflammatory properties, can soothe the gut lining and alleviate nausea, while peppermint has been shown to relax the muscles of the gastrointestinal tract, providing relief from bloating and discomfort. Chamomile not only acts as a mild sedative but also aids digestion by reducing inflammation in the intestines. Incorporating these herbs into daily routines, whether through herbal teas or as culinary ingredients, can enhance digestive wellness and promote a healthy gut environment.

In addition to herbs, prebiotic foods such as garlic, onions, asparagus, and bananas play a significant role in nurturing gut bacteria. These foods are rich in fiber and act as food sources for beneficial gut microbes. By promoting the growth of these probiotics, prebiotics help maintain a balanced gut flora, which is essential for efficient digestion and overall health. Regular consumption of prebiotic foods can help prevent dysbiosis, a condition characterized by an imbalance of gut bacteria that can lead to various digestive disorders and other health issues.

Smoothies can serve as a delicious and effective vehicle for incorporating gut-friendly ingredients into your diet. Ingredients like spinach, avocados, and kefir not only provide essential nutrients but also contribute to gut health through their high fiber content and probiotic properties. Adding anti-inflammatory herbs such as turmeric and cinnamon can enhance the smoothie's benefits, making it a powerful concoction for those looking to support their digestive health. Experimenting with different combinations of fruits, vegetables, and herbs can lead to tasty recipes that nourish the gut while supporting fitness goals.

For individuals dealing with specific digestive disorders such as irritable bowel syndrome (IBS), certain herbal remedies can offer relief. Herbs like fennel and licorice root have demonstrated effectiveness in alleviating symptoms associated with IBS, including gas, bloating, and cramping. Moreover, detoxifying herbs such as dandelion and milk thistle support liver function, which is intricately linked to gut health. Utilizing these herbs in conjunction with a balanced diet can provide a comprehensive approach to managing digestive issues and enhancing overall gut health, paving the way for a healthier, more vibrant life.

CHAPTER 5

"Introduction to Detoxifying Herbs"

What Are Detoxifying Herbs?

Detoxifying herbs play a crucial role in the realm of gut health, offering a natural and effective means to cleanse and rejuvenate the digestive system. These herbs are known for their ability to support the body's detoxification processes, aiding in the elimination of harmful toxins and promoting overall digestive wellness. They can enhance liver function, stimulate bile production, and improve nutrient absorption, which are all vital for maintaining a healthy gut environment. Understanding the properties and benefits of detoxifying herbs is essential for anyone looking to optimize their health through natural means.

Among the various detoxifying herbs, certain ones stand out for their potent effects on gut health. Milk thistle, for instance, is renowned for its liver-protective qualities, thanks to its active compound, silymarin. This herb not only aids in detoxification but also supports the regeneration of liver cells, ensuring that the organ functions efficiently. Dandelion root is another powerful herb that promotes bile flow, facilitating digestion and fat metabolism. Its natural diuretic properties also help in flushing out toxins, making it an excellent addition to any detox regimen.

Incorporating these herbs into your daily routine can be achieved through various methods, one of the most popular being herbal teas. Herbal teas made from detoxifying herbs like peppermint, ginger, and chamomile can provide soothing effects on the digestive tract while simultaneously supporting detoxification. Additionally, these teas can serve as a gentle introduction to herbal remedies for those grappling with digestive disorders such as irritable bowel syndrome (IBS). The warm infusion not only aids in digestion but also promotes relaxation, further enhancing gut health.

A holistic approach to gut health also includes the integration of prebiotic foods alongside detoxifying herbs. Foods rich in prebiotics, such as garlic, onions, and bananas, help nourish the beneficial gut flora, creating a balanced microbiome. This combination of detoxifying herbs and prebiotic foods can lead to improved digestion, reduced inflammation, and enhanced overall gut function. By understanding the synergistic effects of these elements, individuals can create a more comprehensive strategy for gut health.

For those seeking to maximize the benefits of detoxifying herbs, incorporating them into gut-friendly smoothie recipes can be an effective strategy. Smoothies made with ingredients like spinach, kale, and fruits combined with detoxifying herbs provide a nutrient-dense option that supports both cleansing and nourishment. By blending these ingredients, individuals can easily consume a concentrated dose of vitamins, minerals, and antioxidants, further promoting digestive health. Embracing detoxifying herbs as part of a broader dietary approach empowers individuals to take charge of their gut health and overall well-being.

The Science Behind Detoxification

Detoxification is a fundamental process that the body undergoes to eliminate toxins and waste products, maintaining overall health and wellness. The liver, kidneys, skin, and gastrointestinal tract play critical roles in this process, working synergistically to filter and expel harmful substances. Understanding the science behind detoxification highlights the importance of supporting these organs with nutrient-dense foods, particularly herbs known for their detoxifying properties. By focusing on gut health, we can enhance the body's natural cleansing mechanisms and promote a balanced microbiome.

Herbs possess unique phytochemicals that contribute to their detoxifying effects. Compounds such as flavonoids, alkaloids, and terpenes found in various herbs can stimulate liver enzymes that facilitate the conversion of toxins into water-soluble compounds, allowing for easier excretion. For instance, herbs like milk thistle and dandelion root are renowned for their ability to support liver function, while burdock root aids in the elimination of waste through the kidneys. Incorporating these herbs into daily routines, whether through teas or culinary applications, can significantly bolster the body's detoxification pathways.

Moreover, the gut microbiota plays a pivotal role in detoxification and overall digestive health. A balanced gut flora enhances the breakdown and removal of toxins from the digestive tract. Prebiotic foods, such as garlic, onions, and asparagus, serve as nourishment for beneficial gut bacteria, promoting their growth and activity. This symbiotic relationship not only supports detoxification but also helps mitigate inflammation and improve nutrient absorption. By focusing on a diet rich in prebiotics and fiber, individuals can foster a thriving microbiome that aids in detoxification.

In addition to herbs and prebiotic foods, herbal teas are an effective way to promote digestive wellness and support detoxification processes. Herbal infusions made from ingredients like ginger, peppermint, and chamomile can soothe digestive discomfort while simultaneously aiding in detoxification. These teas help stimulate digestion and increase bile production, further enhancing the body's ability to process and eliminate toxins. Regular consumption of gut-friendly herbal teas can create a routine that supports both detoxification and overall digestive health.

Individuals dealing with digestive disorders, such as IBS, can particularly benefit from targeted herbal remedies that support detoxification and gut health. Anti-inflammatory herbs, including turmeric and licorice root, can alleviate symptoms while promoting a balanced digestive environment. Combining these herbs with gut-friendly smoothie recipes that incorporate fruits, vegetables, and probiotics can create a powerful synergistic effect, enhancing both detoxification and overall digestive function. By prioritizing these approaches, fitness and health enthusiasts can achieve a healthier gut and a more effective detoxification process.

How to Incorporate Herbs into Your Diet

Incorporating herbs into your diet is a powerful way to enhance gut health and overall wellness. Herbs have been used for centuries in traditional medicine, and modern research supports their efficacy in promoting digestive health. One of the simplest methods to introduce herbs into your meals is by using fresh herbs in cooking. Basil, cilantro, and parsley can be added to salads, soups, and main dishes to not only elevate flavor but also provide essential nutrients and digestive benefits. Cooking with herbs like oregano and thyme can also impart anti-inflammatory properties, helping to soothe digestive discomfort and support overall gut function.

Herbal teas are another excellent avenue for integrating herbs into your diet, particularly for those focused on digestive wellness. Teas made from ginger, peppermint, and chamomile can help alleviate symptoms of bloating, gas, and nausea. These soothing beverages are easy to prepare and can be enjoyed throughout the day. Additionally, herbal teas can serve as a comforting ritual, allowing you to take a moment for yourself while promoting gut health. For maximum benefits, consider steeping fresh herbs in hot water and adding a squeeze of lemon for an extra detoxifying boost.

For those interested in prebiotic foods, incorporating herbs such as garlic and onion into your meals can be particularly beneficial. These herbs not only add depth to your dishes but also promote the growth of healthy gut flora. Prebiotics are essential for maintaining a balanced microbiome, which is crucial for digestion and overall health. By combining these herbs with fiber-rich foods like whole grains, fruits, and vegetables, you can create gut-friendly meals that support digestive wellness and enhance nutrient absorption.

Smoothies are a versatile way to harness the power of herbs while enjoying a nutrient-packed meal. Adding herbs like spinach, kale, or mint to your smoothies can enhance their nutritional profile and provide anti-inflammatory benefits. Additionally, herbs like fennel can aid digestion and provide a refreshing flavor. Experimenting with different combinations of fruits, vegetables, and herbs can lead to delicious blends that not only please the palate but also support your gut health.

Finally, for those dealing with specific digestive issues such as Irritable Bowel Syndrome (IBS), herbal remedies can offer relief. Herbs like slippery elm and marshmallow root are known for their soothing properties, helping to coat the digestive tract and reduce irritation. Incorporating these herbs into your diet, whether through tinctures, capsules, or teas, can be an effective strategy for managing symptoms. Moreover, seeking guidance from a healthcare professional can help tailor your approach, ensuring that you maximize the benefits of herbs in your journey toward digestive wellness.

CHAPTER 6

" Herbal Teas for Digestive Wellness"

Benefits of Herbal Teas

Herbal teas have gained considerable attention for their myriad benefits, particularly in the realm of gut health. For fitness enthusiasts and health-conscious individuals, these beverages serve not merely as refreshing drinks but as potent allies in promoting digestive wellness. Infused with a variety of herbs, herbal teas can aid in soothing digestive discomfort, reducing inflammation, and supporting overall gut function. This makes them an essential component of any holistic approach to health and wellness.

One of the most significant advantages of herbal teas is their ability to promote digestion. Ingredients such as peppermint and ginger are well-known for their digestive properties, stimulating the production of digestive enzymes and bile. This enhancement in digestion can alleviate symptoms such as bloating and gas, which are common complaints among fitness enthusiasts who may experience these issues due to dietary changes or increased physical activity. Regular consumption of these herbal infusions can lead to improved nutrient absorption and a more robust gut function.

Inflammation is a common underlying factor in many digestive disorders, and herbal teas can play a critical role in mitigating this issue. Herbs like chamomile and turmeric possess anti-inflammatory properties that can help soothe the gut lining and reduce irritation. For individuals dealing with conditions such as irritable bowel syndrome (IBS) or other inflammatory gut disorders, incorporating these teas into their daily routine can provide significant relief. The calming effects of these herbs not only contribute to gut health but also promote overall well-being by reducing stress and anxiety, which are often linked to digestive issues.

Moreover, herbal teas can serve as a natural source of prebiotics, which are essential for maintaining a healthy gut flora balance. Ingredients like dandelion root and licorice root provide nourishment for beneficial gut bacteria, supporting their growth and activity. A healthy microbiome is crucial for optimal digestion, immune function, and even mental health. By integrating herbal teas rich in prebiotic properties into a daily regimen, fitness and health enthusiasts can foster a thriving intestinal environment, enhancing their overall health and vitality.

Finally, the versatility of herbal teas allows for creative incorporation into various health routines. They can be enjoyed hot or cold and used as a base for gut-friendly smoothies or detoxifying drinks. For those looking to cleanse their gut, herbal teas can be an effective tool when paired with a diet rich in whole foods and other detoxifying herbs. This holistic approach not only aids in cleansing but also ensures that individuals are equipping their bodies with the necessary tools to maintain optimal digestive health long-term. Embracing herbal teas as part of a comprehensive gut health strategy can lead to transformative benefits for those committed to their fitness and wellness journeys.

Key Herbs for Digestive Health

Herbal medicine has long been recognized for its ability to support digestive health, offering a natural approach to various gastrointestinal issues. Several key herbs possess potent properties that can enhance gut function, alleviate discomfort, and promote overall wellness. Understanding these herbs and their specific benefits can empower individuals on their journey to better digestive health. From soothing inflammation to balancing gut flora, the right herbs can play a crucial role in fostering a healthier digestive system.

Ginger is one of the most well-known herbs in digestive health, renowned for its anti-inflammatory and carminative properties. It aids in reducing nausea and bloating, making it an excellent choice for those suffering from digestive discomfort. Incorporating ginger into herbal teas or smoothies can enhance flavor while providing significant relief. Additionally, ginger stimulates the production of digestive enzymes, which can improve the breakdown and absorption of nutrients, thus supporting optimal gut function.

Peppermint is another powerful herb that can contribute to digestive wellness. Its menthol content provides a calming effect on the gastrointestinal tract, which can help alleviate symptoms of irritable bowel syndrome (IBS) and other digestive disorders. Peppermint tea is a popular remedy for easing cramping and gas, while its aromatic properties can enhance digestion by promoting bile flow. Regular consumption of peppermint can also help balance gut flora, making it a versatile herb for maintaining digestive health.

Turmeric, with its active component curcumin, stands out for its potent anti-inflammatory properties. This herb not only supports gut health by reducing inflammation but also plays a role in protecting the gut lining from damage. Turmeric can be easily incorporated into meals or taken as a supplement, providing a natural way to combat digestive discomfort and promote healing. Its antioxidant properties further enhance its effectiveness, making it a valuable addition to any digestive health regimen.

Finally, incorporating prebiotic foods such as garlic and onions can significantly benefit gut flora balance. These foods nourish beneficial bacteria, fostering a thriving microbiome essential for digestive health. When combined with herbal remedies, the effects can be amplified, creating a holistic approach to gut wellness. Additionally, herbal blends that include chamomile and fennel can be excellent choices for soothing digestion and reducing inflammation. By integrating these key herbs and prebiotic foods into daily routines, individuals can cultivate a healthier gut and experience the long-term benefits of improved digestive health.

Recipes for Digestive Herbal Teas

Herbal teas have long been celebrated for their therapeutic properties, particularly in supporting digestive health. Crafting the right blend of herbs can not only enhance digestion but also promote a balanced gut flora, which is essential for overall wellness. In this section, we will explore several recipes for herbal teas that can aid in digestion, reduce inflammation, and assist in detoxifying the gut. These recipes are designed for health-conscious individuals seeking natural solutions to enhance their digestive wellness.

One potent recipe includes a combination of peppermint, ginger, and chamomile. Peppermint is known for its ability to relieve bloating and gas, while ginger acts as a powerful anti-inflammatory agent that can soothe the digestive tract. Chamomile adds a calming effect that can alleviate stress-related digestive issues. To prepare this tea, steep one tablespoon of dried peppermint leaves, one tablespoon of grated fresh ginger, and one tablespoon of dried chamomile flowers in four cups of boiling water for about 10-15 minutes. Strain the mixture and enjoy it warm, preferably after meals to aid in digestion.

Another effective blend features fennel seeds, licorice root, and dandelion root. Fennel seeds are recognized for their ability to reduce symptoms of bloating and gas, while licorice root can help soothe the gut lining and improve overall digestive function. Dandelion root supports liver function, which is crucial for detoxification. To make this tea, combine one teaspoon of fennel seeds, one teaspoon of dried licorice root, and one teaspoon of dried dandelion root in boiling water.

Let it steep for 10 minutes before straining. This tea can be consumed both hot or cold and is particularly beneficial in the morning to kickstart digestion.

For those seeking a more refreshing option, a detoxifying herbal tea using lemon balm, nettle, and green tea could be ideal. Lemon balm is known for its calming properties and can help ease digestive discomfort, while nettle is rich in vitamins and minerals that support gut health. Green tea provides additional antioxidant benefits, promoting overall wellness. To prepare this invigorating blend, steep one tablespoon of dried lemon balm, one tablespoon of dried nettle, and one teaspoon of green tea leaves in hot water for about five minutes. This tea can be enjoyed throughout the day, providing hydration and digestive support.

Lastly, consider a blend that focuses on prebiotic benefits with ingredients like dandelion greens, ginger, and turmeric. Dandelion greens are an excellent source of prebiotics, which nourish beneficial gut bacteria. Ginger and turmeric both possess strong anti-inflammatory properties that can alleviate digestive distress. To create this tea, steep a handful of fresh dandelion greens, one tablespoon of fresh grated ginger, and a teaspoon of turmeric powder in four cups of boiling water. After steeping for 15 minutes, strain and enjoy. This herbal infusion not only promotes gut health but also supports a robust immune system.

Incorporating these herbal tea recipes into your daily routine can significantly enhance your digestive health. Each blend is designed to leverage the unique properties of various herbs, providing a holistic approach to gut wellness. By focusing on natural ingredients, you can create soothing and restorative teas that not only detoxify but also support a balanced gut microbiome. As you explore these recipes, remember that consistency is key; regular consumption can lead to lasting benefits for your digestive system.

CHAPTER 7

"Anti-Inflammatory Herbs for Digestive Health, Understanding Inflammation in the Gut"

Inflammation in the gut is a crucial aspect of overall health that often goes unnoticed until it manifests as discomfort or more severe digestive issues. The gut is not merely a passage for food; it is a complex ecosystem that houses trillions of microorganisms. This microbiome plays a pivotal role in maintaining gut health, aiding digestion, and supporting the immune system. When the balance of this ecosystem is disrupted, inflammation can arise, leading to conditions such as irritable bowel syndrome (IBS), inflammatory bowel disease (IBD), and other digestive disorders. Understanding the underlying mechanisms of gut inflammation is essential for those seeking to implement effective herbal and dietary solutions.

One of the primary drivers of gut inflammation is the consumption of pro-inflammatory foods. Diets high in refined sugars, unhealthy fats, and processed foods can trigger an inflammatory response, disrupting the microbiome balance. In contrast, incorporating anti-inflammatory herbs and nutrient-dense foods can significantly mitigate inflammation. Herbs such as turmeric, ginger, and chamomile have well-documented anti-inflammatory properties that can soothe the digestive tract and promote healing. Additionally, adopting a diet rich in prebiotic foods, such as garlic, onions, and bananas, can nourish beneficial gut bacteria, further aiding in reducing inflammation.

Herbal teas have emerged as a popular and effective means of promoting digestive wellness. Teas made from peppermint, fennel, and licorice root not only provide hydration but also possess properties that can alleviate inflammation and support gut motility. These soothing infusions can be consumed regularly to create a calming effect on the digestive system. Moreover, the ritual of enjoying herbal tea can serve as a mindful practice, encouraging individuals to slow down and pay attention to their body's needs, which is essential for overall digestive health.

Prebiotic foods play an essential role in maintaining gut flora balance, fostering a healthy microbiome that can resist inflammation. Foods high in fiber, such as legumes, whole grains, and certain fruits and vegetables, act as food for beneficial bacteria, promoting their growth and activity. This symbiotic relationship is critical for gut health, as a diverse microbiome can better regulate inflammation and protect against gut-related disorders. Including a variety of prebiotic-rich foods in daily meals can enhance digestive function and contribute to a more resilient gut environment.

For those struggling with IBS and other digestive disorders, exploring herbal remedies can provide significant relief. Specific herbs, such as slippery elm and marshmallow root, have mucilaginous properties that can coat and protect the gut lining, reducing inflammation and irritation. Furthermore, adopting gut-friendly smoothie recipes that blend anti-inflammatory ingredients with prebiotic foods can create a potent tool for gut cleansing and recovery. These smoothies not only offer a quick and nutritious option but also serve as a delicious way to incorporate healing herbs and foods into a daily routine, fostering long-term digestive health and wellness.

Top Anti-Inflammatory Herbs

Inflammation plays a significant role in various digestive disorders, contributing to discomfort, bloating, and other gastrointestinal issues. Incorporating anti-inflammatory herbs into your diet can be a powerful strategy for promoting gut health and overall well-being. These herbs not only help reduce inflammation but also support digestion, enhance nutrient absorption, and provide a range of additional health benefits. Understanding the top anti-inflammatory herbs and their properties can empower individuals seeking to improve their gut health through natural means.

Turmeric, often hailed as a super herb, contains curcumin, a compound known for its potent anti-inflammatory effects. Studies have shown that curcumin can help reduce inflammatory markers in the body, making it an excellent addition to any gut-friendly regimen. Incorporating turmeric into your meals or brewing it into a herbal tea can enhance digestive health and alleviate symptoms associated with conditions such as irritable bowel syndrome (IBS). Its vibrant color and warm flavor also make it a versatile ingredient for various dishes, from smoothies to soups.

Ginger is another remarkable anti-inflammatory herb that has been used for centuries to aid digestion. Its active compounds, gingerols and shogaols, have demonstrated the ability to reduce inflammation and soothe the digestive tract. Regular consumption of ginger tea can ease nausea and promote gut motility, making it particularly beneficial for those experiencing digestive discomfort. Additionally, ginger can be easily incorporated into your diet through various culinary applications, from stir-fries to baked goods, making it a convenient choice for maintaining gut health.

Boswellia is less commonly known but holds significant promise as an anti-inflammatory herb for gut health. It contains boswellic acids, which have been shown to inhibit the production of inflammatory cytokines. This herb is particularly beneficial for individuals dealing with chronic inflammatory conditions, including inflammatory bowel disease (IBD). Boswellia can be found in supplement form or as a tincture, offering a concentrated option for those looking to harness its potent properties. Including this herb in your health regimen may lead to improved gut health and reduced inflammation.

Lastly, peppermint deserves mention as an effective anti-inflammatory herb that also aids digestion. Its menthol content provides a cooling effect that can help alleviate bloating and discomfort. Peppermint tea is a soothing option for those who experience digestive issues, and its aroma can also stimulate appetite and enhance the overall digestive process. By integrating peppermint into your routine, whether through tea or as an ingredient in dishes, you can support your digestive system while enjoying its refreshing flavor.

Incorporating these top anti-inflammatory herbs into your diet can significantly enhance your gut health journey. From turmeric and ginger to boswellia and peppermint, these herbs offer a range of benefits that extend beyond inflammation reduction. As you explore various herbal teas, prebiotic foods, and gut-friendly recipes, consider how these powerful herbs can complement your efforts in achieving a healthier, more balanced digestive system. Embracing these natural solutions is an empowering step toward a holistic approach to gut health and well-being.

Incorporating These Herbs into Your Diet

Incorporating detoxifying herbs into your diet is an effective strategy for enhancing gut health and overall well-being. A variety of herbs can be easily integrated into daily meals, offering both flavor and health benefits. For instance, herbs like peppermint and ginger can be added to smoothies, salads, or soups. These herbs not only provide a refreshing taste but also contribute to digestive wellness by soothing the stomach and promoting healthy digestion. By making small adjustments to your cooking and eating habits, you can reap the rewards of these powerful plants.

Herbal teas are a convenient and enjoyable way to promote digestive health. Infusions made from chamomile, fennel, and dandelion root can be consumed throughout the day, offering hydration along with gut-friendly properties. Chamomile is known for its calming effects, which can help alleviate digestive discomfort, while fennel acts as a natural carminative, reducing bloating and gas. Incorporating these teas into your routine not only helps in detoxifying your gut but also serves as a soothing ritual that can enhance overall mental well-being.

Prebiotic foods play a crucial role in maintaining a balanced gut flora, and many herbs can serve as effective prebiotics. Garlic, leeks, and onions are examples of herbs that can be easily included in meals to support the growth of beneficial gut bacteria. These ingredients can be used in various dishes, from stir-fries to roasted vegetables, ensuring that your meals are both nutritious and flavorful. By prioritizing these prebiotic-rich herbs, you can create a gut-friendly environment that fosters optimal digestive health.

When dealing with specific digestive disorders such as IBS, certain herbal remedies can offer relief. Herbs like slippery elm and marshmallow root have mucilaginous properties that can soothe the intestinal lining and reduce inflammation. Incorporating these herbs into your diet can be achieved through teas, powders, or capsules, depending on personal preference. Understanding the right dosage and form of these herbs is essential for maximizing their benefits, particularly for those with sensitive digestive systems.

Smoothies are an excellent medium for incorporating various herbs into your diet. By blending ingredients like spinach, kale, and anti-inflammatory herbs such as turmeric and cilantro, you can create a nutrient-dense beverage that supports gut health. Adding a scoop of flaxseeds or chia seeds enhances the fiber content, further promoting digestive regularity. Experimenting with different combinations not only keeps your meals interesting but also ensures that you're consistently nourishing your gut with the healing properties of nature's finest herbs.

CHAPTER 8

"Prebiotic Foods for Gut Flora Balance"

What Are Prebiotics?

Prebiotics are non-digestible food components that play a crucial role in maintaining gut health by promoting the growth and activity of beneficial gut bacteria. Unlike probiotics, which are live microorganisms, prebiotics serve as food for these bacteria, enhancing their ability to flourish in the digestive tract. This symbiotic relationship is essential for optimal gut flora balance, which is vital for overall health and well-being. As fitness and health enthusiasts, understanding the importance of prebiotics can significantly influence your dietary choices and contribute to your fitness goals.

Common sources of prebiotics include a variety of foods rich in dietary fibers, particularly resistant starch and certain oligosaccharides. Foods such as bananas, onions, garlic, leeks, asparagus, and chicory root are excellent prebiotic sources. Incorporating these foods into your diet can enhance gut flora, leading to improved digestion and nutrient absorption. For those interested in herbal remedies, certain herbs also exhibit prebiotic properties, making them valuable additions to your diet. Such herbs can be effectively used in various forms, including teas and supplements, to support digestive health.

The benefits of prebiotics extend beyond promoting gut bacteria growth. They help in producing short-chain fatty acids, which are essential for colon health and have anti-inflammatory properties. This is particularly relevant for individuals dealing with digestive disorders, such as IBS, where inflammation can exacerbate symptoms. By regularly consuming prebiotic-rich foods, you can support your body's natural defenses and create an environment conducive to healing within the gut.

Incorporating prebiotics into your diet can also enhance the effectiveness of probiotics. A healthy balance between probiotics and prebiotics is necessary for achieving optimal gut health. This synergy is often referred to as synbiotics, where the presence of prebiotics enhances the survival and activity of probiotics in the gastrointestinal tract. Creating gut-friendly smoothie recipes that include both prebiotic-rich ingredients and probiotic sources like yogurt or kefir can be an innovative way to support your digestive wellness while enjoying delicious and nutritious beverages.

For those seeking a comprehensive approach to gut health, prebiotics are an indispensable component. They not only support the growth of beneficial bacteria but also contribute to overall digestive health and immune function. By prioritizing prebiotic foods and herbs in your diet, you can take significant steps toward detoxifying your gut and alleviating digestive disorders. Emphasizing the inclusion of prebiotics can lead to a more balanced gut flora, enhancing your overall health and fitness journey.

Benefits of Prebiotics for Gut Health

Prebiotics play a crucial role in maintaining and enhancing gut health, making them an essential component for fitness and health enthusiasts seeking to optimize their digestive systems. These non-digestible fibers serve as food for beneficial gut bacteria, promoting a healthy microbiome. By incorporating prebiotic-rich foods into the diet, individuals can create an environment conducive to the flourishing of these beneficial organisms. This not only aids digestion but also supports overall health, contributing to the body's ability to detoxify and recover from various stresses, particularly after intense workouts.

The consumption of prebiotics has been linked to improved gut flora balance, an essential aspect of digestive wellness. Foods such as garlic, onions, leeks, and asparagus are rich in inulin and other prebiotic fibers that encourage the growth of probiotics. A balanced gut microbiome is vital for efficient nutrient absorption, which is particularly important for those engaged in regular physical activity. Better nutrient absorption translates to enhanced energy levels, improved recovery times, and increased performance during workouts, making prebiotics an indispensable ally for fitness enthusiasts.

In addition to supporting gut flora balance, prebiotics exhibit anti-inflammatory properties that can significantly benefit those suffering from digestive disorders, including Irritable Bowel Syndrome (IBS). By reducing inflammation in the gut, prebiotics can alleviate symptoms such as bloating, gas, and discomfort, allowing individuals to enjoy their meals without the fear of post-meal distress. This relief can lead to more consistent training schedules and improved physical performance, as discomfort from digestive issues can often hinder one's ability to engage fully in workouts.

Furthermore, incorporating prebiotic foods into a daily routine can enhance the efficacy of herbal remedies aimed at digestive health. When combined with anti-inflammatory herbs, such as ginger or turmeric, prebiotics work synergistically to boost the overall effectiveness of these natural treatments. This combination not only aids in cleansing the gut but also supports a more resilient immune system, which is particularly beneficial for those who prioritize fitness and overall well-being.

Finally, the versatility of prebiotic foods allows for creative dietary choices, including gut-friendly smoothie recipes that can easily be integrated into any fitness regimen. Smoothies can serve as an excellent vehicle for blending prebiotic ingredients with other healthful herbs and foods, resulting in delicious and nutrient-dense meals. By embracing the benefits of prebiotics, individuals can foster a healthier gut environment, enhance their detoxification processes, and ultimately support their fitness goals more effectively.

List of Prebiotic Foods

Prebiotic foods play a crucial role in maintaining gut health by serving as nourishment for beneficial gut bacteria. These non-digestible fibers stimulate the growth and activity of probiotics, promoting a balanced microbiome. A diverse and healthy gut flora is essential for optimal digestive function, immune support, and overall well-being. For fitness and health enthusiasts, incorporating prebiotic foods into your diet can enhance the effectiveness of your wellness regimen, particularly when paired with herbal remedies and detoxifying strategies.

One of the most recognized prebiotic foods is chicory root, which is rich in inulin, a type of soluble fiber. Inulin not only encourages the growth of beneficial bacteria such as Bifidobacteria but also supports digestive regularity. Chicory root can be consumed in various forms, including as a coffee substitute or added to smoothies for a nutritional boost. Additionally, this versatile root can be found in many herbal teas, allowing you to enjoy its benefits while hydrating.

Another excellent source of prebiotics is garlic, known for its anti-inflammatory properties and ability to support immune function. Raw garlic contains fructooligosaccharides, which promote the growth of healthy gut bacteria. Incorporating garlic into your meals can enhance flavor while contributing to gut health. For those who prefer a gentler taste, roasted garlic can be a delicious alternative that still provides prebiotic benefits.

Onions, leeks, and asparagus are also notable prebiotic foods. They contain a variety of fibers, including inulin and fructooligosaccharides, that support gut flora balance. These foods can be easily added to salads, stir-fries, or soups, making them accessible options for anyone looking to improve their digestive wellness. Asparagus, in particular, is not only a prebiotic powerhouse but also offers a wealth of vitamins and minerals that contribute to general health.

Finally, bananas, specifically when they are slightly green, are an excellent source of resistant starch, which acts as a prebiotic. This unique carbohydrate resists digestion and ferments in the gut, providing nourishment for beneficial bacteria. Enjoying a banana as a snack or incorporating it into smoothies can be a simple yet effective way to enhance your gut health. By integrating these prebiotic foods into your diet, you can create a solid foundation for a healthy gut microbiome, complementing your overall fitness and health goals.

CHAPTER 9

"Gut-Friendly Smoothie Recipes"

The Role of Smoothies in Gut Health

Smoothies have emerged as a popular tool for enhancing gut health, offering a convenient and delicious way to incorporate a variety of beneficial ingredients into one's diet. For fitness and health enthusiasts, smoothies can serve as a powerful ally in promoting digestive wellness, particularly when they are crafted with a focus on gut-friendly ingredients. By combining fruits, vegetables, herbs, and other nutritious elements, smoothies can provide essential nutrients that support gut function and overall health, making them an ideal choice for those seeking to optimize their digestive systems.

The composition of smoothies allows for the incorporation of prebiotic foods, which play a crucial role in maintaining a balanced gut flora. Ingredients such as bananas, oats, and certain types of fibers are known to act as prebiotics, feeding the beneficial bacteria in the gut. This balance is vital for a healthy digestive system, as it encourages the growth of probiotics, which can improve digestion, enhance nutrient absorption, and support immune function. By regularly including prebiotic-rich ingredients in smoothies, individuals can actively contribute to the establishment and maintenance of a thriving gut microbiome.

In addition to prebiotics, smoothies can be enhanced with anti-inflammatory herbs that support digestive health. Turmeric, ginger, and peppermint are notable examples that can be easily blended into smoothies. These herbs not only add flavor but also possess properties that can reduce inflammation in the gastrointestinal tract. This is particularly beneficial for those suffering from conditions like irritable bowel syndrome (IBS) or other digestive disorders, as they can help alleviate symptoms and promote a more comfortable digestive experience. Incorporating these herbs into daily smoothies can transform them into potent remedies for maintaining gut health.

Moreover, smoothies offer an excellent platform for detoxifying herbs, which can aid in cleansing the gut and promoting overall digestive health. Ingredients such as dandelion greens, cilantro, and parsley are rich in antioxidants and can support the liver and digestive system in eliminating toxins. By blending these detoxifying herbs into a smoothie, individuals can create a nutrient-dense drink that not only refreshes but also contributes to gut cleansing. This is especially relevant for those looking to reset their digestive systems while enjoying a flavorful and satisfying beverage.

Lastly, the versatility of smoothies means that they can be tailored to meet individual dietary needs and preferences. For those with specific digestive challenges, such as lactose intolerance or gluten sensitivity, smoothies can be easily adjusted to include suitable alternatives that do not compromise gut health. By experimenting with different combinations of fruits, vegetables, and herbs, fitness and health enthusiasts can create personalized smoothies that not only taste great but also support their gut health goals. This adaptability makes smoothies an invaluable addition to any health-focused regimen, particularly for those committed to improving their digestive wellness through natural means.

Key Ingredients for Gut-Friendly Smoothies

Key ingredients for gut-friendly smoothies play a crucial role in promoting digestive health and overall wellness. When crafting a smoothie aimed at enhancing gut function, it is essential to incorporate a balance of fiber-rich fruits and vegetables, prebiotic foods, and anti-inflammatory herbs. Each ingredient contributes to a synergistic effect that not only supports gut flora but also aids in detoxification processes, making these smoothies a powerful ally in your health regimen.

Fruits such as bananas, apples, and berries are excellent choices for a gut-friendly smoothie. Bananas are high in potassium and serve as a natural prebiotic, feeding beneficial gut bacteria. Apples, particularly with their skin, provide pectin, a soluble fiber that enhances digestion and promotes regularity. Berries, rich in antioxidants and fiber, help reduce inflammation in the gut while also providing a burst of flavor. Incorporating these fruits not only enhances the nutritional profile of the smoothie but also ensures a naturally sweet taste without the need for added sugars.

Vegetables like spinach, kale, and cucumber are invaluable additions to any gut-friendly smoothie. Leafy greens are packed with vitamins, minerals, and fiber, which support detoxification and provide essential nutrients for overall health. Spinach and kale are also rich in magnesium, a mineral that plays a key role in digestive health. Cucumbers add hydration and are low in calories, making them an excellent choice for those looking to maintain a healthy weight while supporting gut function. The combination of these vegetables can create a nutrient-dense base for your smoothie.

Incorporating prebiotic foods such as oats, flaxseeds, or chia seeds can significantly enhance the gut-supportive qualities of your smoothie. Oats are a great source of soluble fiber and can help regulate bowel movements while promoting the growth of beneficial bacteria. Flaxseeds and chia seeds are not only high in fiber but also provide omega-3 fatty acids, which are known for their anti-inflammatory properties. These ingredients help to maintain a healthy balance of gut flora, fostering an environment conducive to digestive wellness.

Finally, adding herbal elements such as ginger, peppermint, or turmeric can elevate the gut-friendly profile of your smoothie. Ginger is renowned for its ability to soothe digestive discomfort and reduce inflammation, making it a valuable ingredient for those with sensitive stomachs. Peppermint can help relieve bloating and improve overall digestion, while turmeric provides powerful anti-inflammatory benefits. These herbs not only enhance the flavor of your smoothie but also contribute to a holistic approach to gut health, making your drink not just a meal but a strategic tool in your wellness journey.

Delicious Smoothie Recipes

Delicious smoothies can be a powerful ally in promoting gut health, especially when infused with detoxifying herbs and nutrient-rich ingredients. These beverages not only serve as a convenient meal or snack option but also provide a concentrated source of vitamins, minerals, and antioxidants essential for maintaining a healthy digestive system. By incorporating gut-friendly ingredients into your smoothie recipes, you can support your body's natural cleansing processes while enjoying a delicious treat that satisfies your taste buds.

One of the cornerstone ingredients in gut-friendly smoothies is spinach, a leafy green rich in fiber and prebiotics that foster the growth of beneficial gut flora. Combine spinach with banana, which adds natural sweetness and potassium, and a tablespoon of chia seeds for added fiber and omega-3 fatty acids. Blend these together with unsweetened almond milk or coconut water, and you have a refreshing, nutrient-dense smoothie that promotes digestive health. The fiber from both the spinach and chia seeds aids in maintaining regular bowel movements, while the potassium in bananas helps regulate electrolyte balance.

Herbs like ginger and turmeric are celebrated for their anti-inflammatory properties and can be seamlessly integrated into smoothie recipes. A ginger-turmeric smoothie can be both invigorating and soothing for the gut. Start with a base of coconut milk or yogurt, which provides probiotics beneficial for gut flora balance. Add fresh ginger and turmeric root or their powdered forms, along with a squeeze of lemon juice and a dash of black pepper to enhance absorption of curcumin, the active compound in turmeric. This combination not only enhances digestive function but also supports the body in reducing inflammation, making it ideal for those experiencing digestive discomfort.

For those seeking a sweet and satisfying option, a berry smoothie with detoxifying herbs can be both delicious and nutritious. Blend a mix of blueberries, strawberries, and raspberries, which are high in antioxidants and fiber, with a handful of kale or Swiss chard. Incorporate a tablespoon of flaxseed or hemp seeds for additional omega-3s. To boost the detoxifying effects, consider adding dandelion greens or milk thistle, both of which support liver function and detoxification. This vibrant smoothie not only tastes great but also promotes gut health by providing essential nutrients and antioxidants that combat oxidative stress.

Lastly, a creamy avocado and probiotic-rich yogurt smoothie can serve as a perfect post-workout recovery drink. Avocado is a great source of healthy fats and fiber, which helps in keeping you satiated while also promoting gut health. Blend ripe avocado with plain yogurt, a splash of lime juice, and a handful of mint or basil for a refreshing twist. This smoothie not only aids in digestion but also provides a rich source of probiotics that enhance gut flora diversity. By incorporating these delicious smoothie recipes into your diet, you can enjoy flavorful and nourishing options that support your journey to optimal gut health.

CHAPTER 10

" Herbal Remedies for IBS and Digestive Disorders"

Understanding IBS and Common Digestive Disorders

Irritable Bowel Syndrome (IBS) is a common yet often misunderstood digestive disorder affecting millions worldwide. Characterized by symptoms such as abdominal pain, bloating, gas, and altered bowel habits, IBS can significantly impact an individual's quality of life. Understanding the intricacies of IBS is crucial, particularly for those invested in fitness and health, as it underscores the importance of gut health in overall well-being. As the gut is often referred to as the "second brain," its proper functioning is essential for nutrient absorption, immune response, and mental health.

In addition to IBS, various digestive disorders may affect individuals, such as inflammatory bowel disease (IBD), celiac disease, and gastroesophageal reflux disease (GERD). Each of these conditions presents unique challenges and symptoms that can disrupt daily activities. For health enthusiasts, recognizing the signs and symptoms of these disorders is vital, as they may often misconstrue them as mere digestive discomfort rather than indicators of underlying health issues. This understanding not only aids in early intervention but also guides dietary and lifestyle choices that can alleviate symptoms and promote digestive health.

Herbs play a significant role in managing IBS and other digestive disorders. Anti-inflammatory herbs like ginger, turmeric, and peppermint have shown promise in easing digestive discomfort and reducing inflammation in the gut. Incorporating these herbs into daily routines, whether through herbal teas or culinary applications, can provide soothing effects. Additionally, specific herbal remedies tailored for IBS, such as fennel and chamomile, can help alleviate symptoms and restore gut balance. For fitness enthusiasts, integrating these herbs into their nutrition regimen can enhance recovery and overall digestive wellness.

Prebiotic foods are another essential aspect of gut health, particularly for those seeking to maintain a balanced gut flora. Foods rich in prebiotics, such as garlic, onions, and bananas, nourish beneficial gut bacteria, promoting a healthy microbiome. A balanced microbiome is crucial for optimal digestion and immune function, making these foods an integral part of any health-focused diet. For those looking to optimize their gut health, incorporating prebiotic foods alongside anti-inflammatory herbs can create a synergistic effect that supports digestive wellness.

Finally, gut-friendly smoothie recipes can serve as a delicious and nutritious way to combine various herbs, prebiotics, and other gut-supporting ingredients. By blending together ingredients such as spinach, kefir, and ground flaxseed, individuals can create smoothies that are not only enjoyable but also packed with nutrients that promote gut health. Detoxifying herbs can further enhance these recipes, aiding in cleansing and revitalizing the digestive system. Adopting a holistic approach that includes understanding IBS and other digestive disorders while utilizing herbal solutions can lead to improved gut health and overall vitality.

Effective Herbal Remedies

In the pursuit of optimal gut health, herbal remedies have emerged as powerful allies in the detoxification process. Many herbs possess unique properties that not only support digestive function but also enhance overall well-being. Incorporating these herbs into your daily routine can help alleviate digestive issues, reduce inflammation, and promote a balanced gut microbiome. It is essential to recognize the specific benefits of various herbs and how they can be effectively integrated into a holistic approach to gut health.

One of the most revered herbs for digestive wellness is ginger. Known for its anti-inflammatory and antioxidant properties, ginger can help soothe the digestive tract, reducing symptoms of nausea and bloating. Incorporating fresh ginger into herbal teas or smoothies can serve as a delicious and effective means of enhancing digestion. Additionally, peppermint is another remarkable herb that can ease digestive discomfort. Its menthol component relaxes the muscles of the gastrointestinal tract, making it particularly beneficial for individuals suffering from irritable bowel syndrome (IBS) or other digestive disorders.

Turmeric, with its active compound curcumin, is celebrated for its potent anti-inflammatory effects. Regular consumption of turmeric can help combat inflammation in the gut and support the healing of the digestive lining. This herb can be easily added to meals or brewed into teas, making it accessible for anyone looking to improve their gut health. Furthermore, dandelion root is often overlooked but is a powerful prebiotic that feeds beneficial gut bacteria, supporting a balanced microbiome. Its ability to stimulate bile production also aids in the digestion of fats, making it a valuable addition to any gut-friendly regimen.

Herbal teas play a significant role in promoting digestive wellness. Blends that include chamomile, fennel, and licorice root can provide calming effects on the digestive system, helping to relieve discomfort and promote relaxation. These teas can be enjoyed after meals to facilitate digestion and support gut health. Additionally, the inclusion of prebiotic foods such as garlic, onions, and asparagus can further nourish beneficial gut flora, enhancing the effectiveness of herbal remedies and contributing to a more balanced digestive environment.

For those facing more severe digestive disorders, targeted herbal remedies can offer significant relief. Herbs like slippery elm and marshmallow root are known for their soothing properties, coating the digestive tract and reducing irritation. These herbs can be particularly useful for individuals suffering from IBS or inflammatory bowel diseases. By understanding the unique properties of these herbal remedies and their role in gut health, fitness enthusiasts and health-conscious individuals can take proactive steps toward achieving optimal digestive wellness through natural means.

How to Use Herbs for Symptom Relief

Incorporating herbs into your daily routine can significantly enhance symptom relief for various digestive issues. Herbs are not just flavorful additions to meals; they are powerful allies that can support gut health through their anti-inflammatory, antimicrobial, and soothing properties. To effectively use herbs for symptom relief, it is essential to understand their specific benefits and how to integrate them into your diet. Knowledge of the right herbs and their applications can empower individuals to manage their gut health more proactively.

One of the most common uses of herbs for digestive wellness is through herbal teas. Teas made from ingredients like peppermint, ginger, and chamomile can alleviate symptoms such as bloating, gas, and general discomfort. Peppermint tea is particularly effective at relaxing the muscles of the gastrointestinal tract, which can help relieve cramps and spasms. Ginger tea, on the other hand, is renowned for its ability to reduce nausea and improve digestion. Regularly sipping these soothing teas can become a cornerstone of a gut-friendly lifestyle, promoting overall digestive health.

In addition to herbal teas, incorporating anti-inflammatory herbs into your meals can offer significant relief from digestive disorders. Turmeric, with its active compound curcumin, is well-known for its potent anti-inflammatory properties. Adding turmeric to soups, smoothies, or even rice dishes can not only enhance flavor but also provide a powerful boost to your gut health. Similarly, herbs such as oregano and thyme possess antimicrobial properties that can help balance gut flora and combat harmful bacteria. These herbs can be easily included in everyday cooking, making them an accessible option for those seeking symptom relief.

Prebiotic foods play a vital role in maintaining a balanced gut microbiome, and certain herbs can complement these efforts. Incorporating garlic and onion into your diet not only adds flavor but also serves as a source of prebiotics, which nourish beneficial gut bacteria. Additionally, incorporating herbs like dandelion and chicory root into salads or smoothies can enhance fiber intake, further supporting gut flora balance. Understanding how to pair these herbs with prebiotic foods can create a synergistic effect that optimizes gut health.

For those dealing with more specific digestive disorders such as IBS, targeted herbal remedies can provide substantial relief. Herbs like fennel and marshmallow root have been traditionally used to alleviate symptoms of IBS, such as abdominal pain and bloating. Fennel seeds can be chewed or brewed into a tea, while marshmallow root can be taken in capsule form or as a tea to soothe the gut lining. Crafting gut-friendly smoothies that include these herbs alongside fruits and vegetables can create a delicious and healing beverage that supports digestive wellness. As you explore the integration of herbs into your diet, remember to pay attention to how your body responds, allowing for personalization of your approach to symptom relief.

CHAPTER 11

" Detoxifying Herbs for Gut Cleansing"

The Need for Gut Cleansing

The need for gut cleansing has gained significant attention in recent years, particularly among fitness and health enthusiasts seeking to optimize their well-being. A well-functioning digestive system is essential not only for nutrient absorption but also for overall health. The gut plays a critical role in immune function, mental health, and inflammation regulation. Therefore, regularly cleansing the gut can enhance these functions, leading to improved physical performance and general vitality.

Modern lifestyles, characterized by processed foods, stress, and environmental toxins, contribute to the accumulation of harmful substances in the gut. These factors can disrupt the delicate balance of gut flora, leading to dysbiosis, which has been associated with various digestive disorders, including irritable bowel syndrome (IBS). By incorporating gut-cleansing practices, such as dietary adjustments and the use of specific herbs, individuals can support their body's natural detoxification processes, promoting a healthier and more balanced gastrointestinal environment.

Herbal teas have emerged as a popular choice for those looking to improve digestive wellness. Ingredients such as ginger, peppermint, and chamomile are not only soothing but also possess anti-inflammatory properties that can alleviate digestive discomfort. These teas can stimulate digestion, reduce bloating, and support gut motility. For those interested in a more holistic approach, integrating these herbal infusions into daily routines can serve as a gentle yet effective method for cleansing the gut and enhancing overall digestive function.

Prebiotic foods play a pivotal role in maintaining a healthy gut flora balance. Foods rich in prebiotics, such as garlic, onions, and bananas, provide nourishment for beneficial bacteria, helping to restore and maintain a diverse microbiome. When combined with detoxifying herbs, these foods can create a synergistic effect, promoting optimal gut health. By prioritizing prebiotic-rich foods along with cleansing herbs, fitness enthusiasts can foster a resilient digestive system that supports their active lifestyles.

In summary, the need for gut cleansing is paramount for anyone committed to fitness and health. By recognizing the importance of a clean and balanced gut, individuals can harness the power of herbal remedies, detoxifying foods, and holistic practices. Embracing these strategies not only addresses existing digestive issues but also acts as a preventive measure, ensuring long-term health and well-being. By making informed choices about gut health, fitness enthusiasts can achieve their wellness goals while enjoying the benefits of a vibrant and resilient digestive system.

Top Detoxifying Herbs

Detoxifying herbs have long been revered for their ability to support gut health and overall wellness. For fitness and health enthusiasts, understanding the benefits of these herbs can enhance your dietary regimen and promote a balanced digestive system. The power of detoxifying herbs lies in their natural compounds that assist in eliminating toxins, reducing inflammation, and supporting the growth of beneficial gut flora. This subchapter will delve into some of the most effective detoxifying herbs that can be easily incorporated into your daily routine.

Milk thistle is one of the foremost herbs recognized for its detoxifying properties. Its active compound, silymarin, plays a crucial role in protecting liver cells and promoting the regeneration of liver tissue. A healthy liver is essential for effective detoxification, as it processes and filters toxins from the body. Incorporating milk thistle into your herbal tea blends or consuming it in supplement form can bolster your liver function, thereby enhancing your gut health. For those looking to optimize their detox regimen, milk thistle is a powerful ally that supports not only liver health but also digestive efficiency.

Another remarkable herb is dandelion root, often overlooked yet immensely beneficial for digestive wellness. Dandelion root acts as a gentle diuretic, aiding in the elimination of excess water and toxins.

Additionally, it stimulates bile production, which is pivotal for the digestion of fats and the absorption of fat-soluble vitamins. With its prebiotic qualities, dandelion root also fosters the growth of beneficial gut bacteria. Adding dandelion root tea to your daily routine can significantly enhance digestive function and contribute to a healthier gut flora balance, making it a staple for those focused on maintaining optimal gut health.

Turmeric, with its active ingredient curcumin, stands out as a powerful anti-inflammatory herb that promotes digestive health. Chronic inflammation can lead to various digestive disorders, including Irritable Bowel Syndrome (IBS) and other gastrointestinal issues. Turmeric's anti-inflammatory properties help reduce inflammation in the gut lining, allowing for improved digestion and nutrient absorption. Incorporating turmeric into smoothies or using it in cooking can provide a flavorful way to harness its benefits. For those seeking natural remedies for digestive disorders, turmeric offers a promising solution that supports both gut health and overall well-being.

Lastly, ginger is renowned for its ability to soothe digestive discomfort and promote gut cleansing. Its natural compounds stimulate gastric motility, helping to ease nausea and support regular bowel movements. Ginger also possesses anti-inflammatory and antioxidant properties that contribute to gut health. Whether consumed as a fresh root, in tea, or as a spice in meals, incorporating ginger into your diet can provide significant digestive benefits. For fitness and health aficionados, ginger serves as an excellent addition to herbal teas and gut-friendly smoothies, enhancing both flavor and health benefits.

In conclusion, the integration of detoxifying herbs such as milk thistle, dandelion root, turmeric, and ginger into your diet can profoundly impact your gut health and overall wellness. By leveraging these powerful herbs, you can support your body's natural detoxification processes, reduce inflammation, and promote a balanced gut microbiome. As you embark on your journey toward improved gut health, consider these herbs not just as supplements, but as essential components of a holistic approach to wellness that embraces the healing power of nature.

Methods for Using Detoxifying Herbs

Detoxifying herbs have long been celebrated for their ability to promote gut health and overall wellness. For fitness and health enthusiasts, incorporating these potent botanicals into daily routines can enhance digestive function and support detoxification processes. Understanding the various methods for using detoxifying herbs is essential for maximizing their benefits. This subchapter will explore effective methods, including herbal teas, tinctures, and food preparations, to harness the power of these natural remedies.

One of the most accessible and popular methods for utilizing detoxifying herbs is through herbal teas. Infusing herbs such as peppermint, ginger, and dandelion into hot water creates a soothing beverage that not only aids digestion but also promotes a sense of relaxation. To prepare an herbal tea, steep the chosen herbs in boiling water for approximately 5 to 10 minutes, allowing their active compounds to be extracted. This method not only provides hydration but also allows the body to absorb beneficial properties that can help alleviate digestive discomfort and reduce inflammation.

Tinctures serve as another effective method for using detoxifying herbs. These concentrated liquid extracts are typically made by soaking herbal material in alcohol or vinegar for several weeks, allowing the extraction of active constituents. Tinctures can be easily added to water or smoothies for a quick and potent dose of herbal benefits. For those dealing with specific digestive issues, such as irritable bowel syndrome (IBS), selecting tinctures that feature anti-inflammatory herbs like turmeric or chamomile can provide targeted relief and support gut health.

Incorporating detoxifying herbs directly into meals is a practical approach that not only adds flavor but also enhances nutritional value. Herbs such as cilantro, parsley, and fennel can be added to salads, soups, and smoothies to improve digestion and promote gut flora balance. Additionally, pairing herbs with prebiotic foods, such as garlic or onions, can create a synergistic effect that further supports the growth of beneficial gut bacteria. This integration of herbs into everyday meals encourages a holistic approach to gut health and detoxification.

For those seeking a refreshing and nutrient-dense option, gut-friendly smoothie recipes can be an excellent vehicle for detoxifying herbs.

Blending ingredients such as spinach, avocado, and ginger with a liquid base like coconut water or almond milk creates a delicious and nourishing drink. Adding herbs like spirulina or nettle can enhance the detoxifying properties of the smoothie, making it an ideal choice for post-workout recovery or as a meal replacement. This method not only supports digestion but also delivers a powerful dose of vitamins and minerals that promote overall health.

In conclusion, utilizing detoxifying herbs through various methods can significantly enhance gut health and support the body's natural detoxification processes. Whether through herbal teas, tinctures, meal preparations, or smoothies, these methods provide versatile options for fitness and health enthusiasts. By integrating detoxifying herbs into daily routines, individuals can experience improved digestive wellness and a deeper sense of vitality.

CHAPTER 12

"Creating a Personalized Gut Health Plan"

Assessing Your Gut Health

Assessing your gut health is critical in understanding overall wellness and optimizing your fitness journey. The gut microbiome, composed of trillions of microorganisms, plays a pivotal role in digestion, immune function, and even mental health. To effectively assess this vital aspect of your health, it is essential to be aware of the signs and symptoms that indicate imbalance. Common indicators include digestive discomfort, such as bloating, gas, irregular bowel movements, and food intolerances. These symptoms can serve as a signal to evaluate your dietary habits and stress levels, both of which significantly impact gut health.

One effective method for assessing gut health is through dietary observation. Keeping a food diary can reveal patterns and trigger foods that may lead to gastrointestinal distress. This practice not only helps identify potential allergens but also highlights the importance of including gut-friendly foods in your diet. Foods rich in prebiotics, such as garlic, onions, and bananas, are crucial for nurturing beneficial gut flora. Additionally, incorporating anti-inflammatory herbs like turmeric and ginger can help mitigate inflammation and support digestive health, further enhancing your body's ability to absorb nutrients.

Incorporating herbal teas into your daily routine can also serve as a barometer for gut health. Herbal teas, such as peppermint and chamomile, are known for their soothing properties and can help alleviate symptoms of indigestion and bloating. By observing how your body responds to these teas, you can gain insight into your digestive health. Regular consumption of these herbal remedies, combined with mindful eating practices, can significantly enhance your digestive wellness. It is important to note how you feel after consuming these beverages, as positive changes can indicate improvements in gut health.

Furthermore, evaluating your body's response to various foods and herbs is crucial for determining the health of your gut. Keeping track of how you feel after consuming specific meals or herbal supplements can provide valuable information. For instance, a smoothie rich in fiber and prebiotic ingredients may enhance your digestion and overall gut flora balance. Conversely, a lack of regular bowel movements or increased discomfort after meals may indicate an imbalance that requires attention. Tailoring your diet based on these observations can lead to more effective management of gut health.

Lastly, understanding the connection between mental health and gut health is essential for a holistic approach to wellness. Stress and anxiety can negatively impact gut function, exacerbating symptoms of conditions like IBS. Mindfulness practices, along with a diet rich in detoxifying herbs, can support both mental and digestive health. Regularly assessing your gut health through these lenses will not only empower you to make informed dietary choices but also foster a deeper understanding of the intricate relationship between your gut and overall well-being. By prioritizing gut health, you contribute to a more balanced and vibrant lifestyle.

Building Your Herbal and Food Strategy

Building your herbal and food strategy is essential for anyone seeking to enhance gut health and overall well-being. The journey begins with understanding the synergy between herbs and foods that can promote digestive wellness. Focusing on the incorporation of anti-inflammatory herbs, prebiotic foods, and herbal remedies tailored for specific digestive disorders can lay a solid foundation for a healthier gut. This approach not only addresses existing issues but also fosters a proactive stance toward maintaining optimal digestive health.

Herbal teas serve as an excellent entry point into the world of herbal remedies. They can be easily integrated into daily routines and provide a soothing, flavorful way to support digestion. Varieties such as ginger, peppermint, and chamomile not only promote digestive comfort but also help mitigate inflammation. Regular consumption of these herbal teas can encourage healthy gut flora and enhance overall digestive function. By establishing a routine that includes these teas, individuals can create a calming ritual that nourishes the gut while also serving as a moment of mindfulness.

Incorporating anti-inflammatory herbs into meals can significantly impact gut health. Herbs such as turmeric, garlic, and cinnamon contain compounds that combat inflammation and support a balanced digestive environment. These herbs can be easily added to recipes, from soups to smoothies, enriching both flavor and nutritional value. Developing a repertoire of recipes that highlight these herbs ensures that they become a regular part of one's dietary strategy, ultimately promoting healing and balance within the digestive tract.

Prebiotic foods play a critical role in nurturing gut flora balance. Foods such as garlic, onions, asparagus, and bananas are rich in fibers that feed beneficial gut bacteria. By strategically including these foods in meals, individuals can enhance their microbiome health, which is essential for digesting food efficiently and absorbing nutrients effectively. Planning meals that combine prebiotic-rich foods with probiotic sources, such as yogurt or fermented vegetables, can optimize gut health, making it a key component of any health-conscious diet.

Lastly, crafting gut-friendly smoothie recipes can serve as a delicious and nutrient-dense element of your herbal and food strategy. Smoothies can be tailored to incorporate a variety of herbs, fruits, and vegetables that support digestion and provide essential vitamins and minerals. Ingredients such as spinach, avocado, and chia seeds, combined with digestive-supportive herbs like mint or parsley, can create a refreshing and healthful drink. Regularly consuming these smoothies not only contributes to hydration and nutrient intake but also reinforces the commitment to a gut-friendly lifestyle, enhancing overall health and vitality.

Tracking Progress and Adjustments

Tracking progress and making adjustments are essential components of any wellness journey, particularly when it comes to gut health. As individuals embark on a cleanse or detox using herbs, it becomes imperative to monitor the effects of these dietary changes on their overall well-being and digestive function. This involves not only observing physical symptoms but also keeping a detailed record of dietary intake, emotional states, and any notable changes in energy levels. By creating a structured tracking system, individuals can identify patterns that correlate with specific herbs or foods, allowing for more informed decisions regarding their gut health protocol.

The use of a food diary can be particularly beneficial in this context. Documenting daily meals, snacks, and herbal tea consumption will enable individuals to assess how various ingredients influence their digestive wellness. For instance, noting the inclusion of prebiotic foods like garlic, onions, or asparagus alongside specific herbs can help determine their effectiveness in promoting gut flora balance. Additionally, tracking the timing and frequency of herbal remedies for conditions such as IBS can provide insights into their impact on symptom relief. This information is invaluable for making necessary adjustments to improve the overall efficacy of the cleansing process.

In conjunction with dietary tracking, self-assessment is vital. Regularly evaluating one's physical and emotional state can highlight how well the body is responding to the detoxifying herbs in use. For example, if an individual experiences increased bloating or discomfort after introducing a new herbal remedy, it may warrant a reevaluation of its suitability. On the other hand, positive changes such as improved digestion or reduced inflammation should be acknowledged and reinforced. By maintaining an open dialogue with oneself about these experiences, individuals can fine-tune their approach and optimize their gut health strategy.

Moreover, the importance of adaptability cannot be understated. As individuals progress through their cleansing journey, they may discover that certain herbs or foods that initially provided benefits may need to be rotated or replaced due to the body's evolving needs. This is especially relevant when considering the body's capacity for adaptation and potential food sensitivities that may develop. Being prepared to make these adjustments can be the key to sustaining long-term digestive health and preventing any stagnation in progress.

Lastly, seeking professional guidance can further enhance the tracking and adjustment process. Collaborating with a nutritionist or herbalist who specializes in gut health can offer additional insights and personalized recommendations. These experts can assist in interpreting tracking data, suggesting alternative herbs or dietary adjustments, and providing support throughout the cleansing journey. By combining personal tracking efforts with professional advice, individuals can create a robust framework for achieving optimal gut health and overall wellness.

CHAPTER 13

"Maintaining Long-Term Gut Health"

Lifestyle Changes for Gut Health

Lifestyle changes are crucial in enhancing gut health, particularly for those already committed to fitness and overall well-being. A well-rounded approach that incorporates dietary adjustments, regular physical activity, and mindfulness practices can significantly improve digestive function and overall health. By focusing on the integration of herbs and food that promote gut wellness, individuals can create an environment conducive to a thriving microbiome.

Incorporating prebiotic foods into your daily diet is essential for maintaining a balanced gut flora. Foods rich in prebiotics, such as garlic, onions, leeks, asparagus, and bananas, not only nourish beneficial gut bacteria but also enhance their activity. These foods can be easily integrated into meals and snacks, providing both flavor and health benefits. For instance, adding sliced bananas to a morning smoothie or incorporating garlic into savory dishes can promote digestive health while supporting an active lifestyle.

Herbal teas are another powerful tool for promoting digestive wellness.

Varieties such as peppermint, ginger, and chamomile can soothe the digestive tract and alleviate symptoms of discomfort. Establishing a routine of sipping herbal teas throughout the day can serve as a calming ritual, enhancing hydration and providing the added benefits of anti-inflammatory properties found in many herbs. This practice can be particularly beneficial after meals, supporting digestion and helping to prevent bloating or discomfort.

Physical activity is integral to gut health, as regular exercise stimulates the digestive system and promotes the movement of food through the intestines. Engaging in activities such as yoga, which emphasizes breath control and relaxation, can further enhance digestive function. Incorporating a variety of workouts—whether high-intensity interval training, strength training, or low-impact exercises—can contribute to improved gut health and overall well-being. The movement encourages blood flow to the digestive organs, facilitating better nutrient absorption and waste elimination.

Finally, adopting mindful eating practices can make a significant difference in gut health. Taking the time to savor meals, chewing food thoroughly, and avoiding distractions during meals can enhance digestion and improve nutrient uptake. This mindful approach, combined with an emphasis on detoxifying herbs such as dandelion and milk thistle, can foster a healthier gut environment. By incorporating these lifestyle changes, fitness enthusiasts can not only support their gut health but also cultivate a more holistic approach to their overall wellness.

The Role of Stress Management

Stress management plays a crucial role in maintaining optimal gut health, particularly for those devoted to fitness and wellness. The gut-brain axis, a complex communication network linking the gastrointestinal tract and the brain, illustrates how emotional and psychological stressors can directly influence digestive function. Chronic stress can lead to a myriad of gastrointestinal issues, including irritable bowel syndrome (IBS), bloating, and dysbiosis. Therefore, effectively managing stress is essential not only for mental well-being but also for promoting a healthy gut microbiome.

Incorporating stress management techniques can significantly enhance the effectiveness of dietary interventions aimed at improving gut health. Mindfulness practices, such as meditation and yoga, have been shown to reduce stress levels and promote relaxation, which can positively impact digestion. These techniques can help to lower cortisol levels, the hormone associated with stress, thereby fostering a more balanced gut environment. When the body is in a state of calm, it can allocate resources more effectively towards digestion and nutrient absorption, ensuring that the benefits of detoxifying herbs and prebiotic foods are fully realized.

Herbal teas can serve as a dual-purpose tool in stress management and digestive wellness. Certain herbal blends, such as chamomile and peppermint, not only soothe the mind but also possess properties that alleviate digestive discomfort. Incorporating these calming teas into daily routines can create moments of pause and mindfulness, allowing individuals to recharge and refocus. By combining the benefits of herbal teas with a diet rich in anti-inflammatory herbs and gut-friendly foods, individuals can create a holistic approach to their health that addresses both stress and digestive function.

Furthermore, a well-balanced diet that includes prebiotic foods is vital for supporting gut flora balance while also providing a foundation for stress resilience. Foods like garlic, onions, and bananas are known to promote the growth of beneficial gut bacteria, which in turn can influence mood and cognitive function. A diverse gut microbiome has been linked to reduced rates of anxiety and depression, showcasing the intricate relationship between gut health and emotional well-being. By nurturing this balance through both diet and stress management strategies, individuals can enhance their overall health and vitality.

In conclusion, the role of stress management in gut health cannot be understated for those dedicated to fitness and wellness. By recognizing the interplay between stress and the digestive system, health enthusiasts can adopt comprehensive strategies that include mindfulness practices, herbal remedies, and nutrient-rich foods. This multifaceted approach not only aids in detoxifying the gut but also fosters a resilient and thriving digestive system, ultimately leading to enhanced overall health and quality of life.

The Importance of Regular Detoxification

Detoxification is a crucial process that supports the body's ability to eliminate toxins, maintain balance, and promote overall well-being. For individuals invested in fitness and health, regular detoxification is not merely a trend but a foundational practice that enhances physical performance and mental clarity. The digestive system, as a primary point of interaction with the external environment, plays a significant role in this process. By focusing on gut health through detoxifying herbs and foods, one can significantly improve nutrient absorption, reduce inflammation, and promote a thriving microbiome.

Incorporating detoxification into a regular health routine can help mitigate the effects of environmental pollutants, dietary toxins, and stress. Many fitness enthusiasts may experience gastrointestinal discomfort or sluggishness due to high-intensity training, poor dietary choices, or exposure to processed foods. By utilizing herbs known for their detoxifying properties, such as dandelion root, burdock root, and milk thistle, individuals can support liver function and enhance the body's natural detox pathways. This not only aids in recovery but also improves overall energy levels, allowing for better performance in workouts and daily activities.

Herbal teas serve as an excellent vehicle for detoxification, providing hydration and vital nutrients that assist in cleansing the digestive system. Varieties such as peppermint, ginger, and chamomile not only soothe the digestive tract but also possess anti-inflammatory properties that can alleviate symptoms associated with digestive disorders, including IBS. Regular consumption of these teas can promote relaxation and balance in the gut, making them a valuable addition to one's daily health regimen. The ritual of brewing and sipping herbal tea also contributes to mindfulness, enhancing the overall detox experience.

Prebiotic foods play an essential role in maintaining gut flora balance while supporting detoxification. Foods like garlic, onions, and asparagus not only nourish beneficial gut bacteria but also assist in the elimination of harmful toxins. By integrating these prebiotic-rich foods into meals, health-conscious individuals can optimize their gut health, ensuring a robust microbiome that is essential for effective detoxification. A balanced gut flora contributes to enhanced digestion, improved immune function, and even better mood regulation, highlighting the interconnectedness of gut health and overall wellness.

Finally, detoxifying herbs can be combined into gut-friendly smoothie recipes, making them both delicious and nutritious. Ingredients such as kale, spinach, and flaxseeds can be blended with detoxifying herbs to create powerful smoothies that support digestion and boost energy levels. These recipes not only offer convenience but also encourage the consumption of a diverse range of nutrients essential for gut health. By prioritizing regular detoxification through herbs and food, fitness and health enthusiasts can cultivate a resilient gut, paving the way for improved health outcomes and a more vibrant lifestyle.

For over 25 years, I've been selective about the foods I consume, ignoring anyone who tries to convince me that certain questionable foods are "okay." I've tried some of them myself, and they simply didn't deliver the results I was after. It's ironic how people who insist that some foods are harmless often struggle with their health, carrying extra weight as a result. Those are the voices you'll want to tune out.

The truth is the people you surround yourself with have a profound impact on your life. Spend time with ten millionaires, and you'll likely become a millionaire. Surround yourself with ten people who are always struggling financially, and you'll find yourself in a similar place. Hang out with ten people living a healthy, balanced lifestyle, and you'll naturally adopt those habits, too. Break free from anything holding you back and find people who share your vision and goals. This principle applies to anything you want to accomplish in life—choose your influences wisely, and success will follow.

Thank every one of you for taking the time to read my health book, "Gut Health Solutions!"

Your feedback is very important, and it helps other readers discover the benefits of improving their gut health.

Please consider leaving a review and share your thoughts on what you learned in my Gut Health Solutions book. Until then, see you next time.

Your Health Coach, Chris D. Henry

Made in the USA
Columbia, SC
15 September 2025

62051944R00065